CODEH 239

FOUR WHEELS
FIVE CORNERS
Facts of Life in Upcountry Maui

PAUL WOOD

Dead Reckoning Books
Haʻiku, Hawaiʻi

A Dead Reckoning Book
Published by Jungle Press

Copyright © 1996 by Paul Wood

All rights reserved under International and Pan-American
Copyright conventions. No part of this publication may be
reproduced, stored in a retrieval system, or transmitted in any
form or by any means – electronic, mechanical, photocopy,
recording, or any other – except for brief quotations in printed
reviews, without the prior written permission of the author.

Published in the United States by Dead Reckoning Books, an
imprint of Jungle Press, Post Office Box 1058, Makawao,
Hawai'i 96768. (piko@aloha.net) 808-572-3453.

ISBN 0-961443-5-5

All essays reprinted by permission of the *Haleakala Times.*

Book design and production by Paul and Barbara Wood
Graphics by Advertising Services and Production
Front cover illustration by Chris Magee, Noodle Design

Manufactured in the U.S.A.

ACKNOWLEDGMENTS

Barbara, my well-loved wife and insightful editor, helped in so many ways, especially by creating the cover and all the wonderful chapter vignettes.

Chris Magee drew the truck (on the cover) and e-mailed it from a bagel shop in Vancouver to Tyler Morrison in Makawao Ranch Acres. Tamara Hanke of Yellowbird contributed a lot of her talent to this book's production. David Warren offered some critical suggestions that made the cover what it is.

Helen at Advertising Services and Production performed marvels making this book ready for the printer

Lots of folks have helped me write these essays by answering my questions and giving me their valuable time, including Eddie Flotte the illustrator, Sandy at Hanzawa Store, Dick Mayer of MCC, Jozef Smit (who spontaneously cartooned), the esteemed philosopher John Dependahl, Makawao Community Police Officer Kris Dixon, Elizabeth Anderson of the Maui County Planning Department, Roy Smith (who should be running the country), John of Maui Recycling, Glenn "The Weatherman" James.

Judy Ivec has been the most encouraging proofreader a writer could have. I've often drawn on my family for inspiration, especially Jake and Tony.

I frequently hear from people who read my column. They send a note or they e-mail. Or they call. Always encouragement. I was out mowing the grass on the roadside, across the street from the house, and a county truck went roaring past on the curve. A big arm shot out the window and gave me a shaka sign, like one good strike with a hammer. Community. Good.

To mention as most honorable last: Ken and Adrienne Pinsky produce the *Haleakala Times*, in which these essays have all appeared as part of my regular column on page two. Our community is better because they have worked so hard.

"It was reckoned a virtue for a man to take a wife, to bring up his children properly, to deal squarely with his neighbors and his landlord, to engage in some industry such as farming, fishing, house-building, canoe-making, or to raise swine, dogs and fowls."

David Malo
Hawaiian Antiquities

CONTENTS

THE PAST:

THE PRESENT:

EDITORIAL NOTE

These essays are arranged according to the plan of this particular book, not in the order of their original publication. They've all been revised since they first appeared in print.

INTRODUCTION

Dead Bomb Shelter and other timely notices

Everyone in Hawai'i can tell you about the good old days. Everyone knows that this island, Maui, used to be a lot better. Some say it was 200 years ago.

Some say it was 2.

There are as many versions of the good old days as there are people to pretend to remember them. And I'd like you to know about mine:

The Makawao dump closed nearly 4 years ago, and my life has felt a little clogged up ever since.

The Makawao dump! You had to drive down into a gulch to get there, between pineapple fields with their million dagger-like leaves bristling into the Earth-blue air.

The road was so bad you didn't ever want to risk it with a passenger car, though people did it all the time. You always saw at least one old van down there, packed with beer cans and banana trash, the owner parked longways to the mildly frightening community trash heap and pitchforking his waste out the sliding door. You watched rickety trailers back into a slot, weaving on the pivot of a rusted-out Datsun hatchback.

You ran into plenty of trucks, too. Lots of them.

That's where we, the rooted people of Upcountry Maui, used to meet as equals, backing up with all the household poop, careful not to get too close together nor to take up too much space along the ever-shifting shoreline of waste. Neighbor toed the line with neighbor for the same humbling task, in the hot gritty breeze, in the squealing din of the Cat's metal treads as it joggled the startled earth, as the white egrets leaped into the clean sky.

Dumps, like public bathrooms, are truly democratic. No one can cop an attitude at the dump. Nobody's poop is any better than anyone else's poop.

In the old Makawao dump, we'd pass brooms around. Sometimes, some reasonably good scrap lumber or an armload of red ti stalks would go right from one guy's truck into his neighbor's. The good old days.

These days, I recycle.

I wait till no one's around and no one's listening to me mutter and gripe. Alone, I learn the sagging weight of each month's sack of beer bottles. I stagger under it, unseen and insignificant in my own back yard.

I preserve my family's poop – sort it, critique it, revisit it, package it, carry it out to the edge of my lawn at dawn on the appointed day. Strangers come, usually when I'm not looking, and then slink away, taking my sorted poop to someplace I never, ever go.

I wash my dog food cans and save them for weeks. I'm saving the planet. Fine.

I just don't want to be seen doing this in public. I'm not going to get together with a bunch of other guys and stand there, elbow to elbow, recycling. ("What – Mel, you think this is aluminum or what?" "I don't know. Got a magnet?") The whole idea is just too sad.

The Makawao dump was never sad.

I remember meeting one of my Portuguese neighbors there, who complained that the dump was filling up and it was all because of the haoles, the white people from the mainland, all those haoles who don't know what to do with their rubbish. In his mind, all of Maui's troubles, including this problem with the dump, began with one major historical tragedy – Statehood.

He was nostalgic for life before 1959. Others I know are nostalgic for life under the monarchy, before the businessmen/traitors stole the kingdom and gave it to America. Others think life got all screwy back in 1778, when Captain Cook showed up.

We all do it.

We all yearn for some kind of past goodness – or we're nostalgic for a future goodness, or we wish the present was like the way we WISH the present was.

Tut tut tut.

I may be partial to dumps, but I have my limits. I write these essays for a different reasons. I write them in the spirit of the Dead Bomb Shelter sign.

The sign stands over a paving dip in downtown Makawao. It doesn't say the usual thing which would be KEEP LEFT, surrounded by fluorescent-colored tape draped on stanchions made from 1" PVC pipe bolted onto plywood squares, like bad sculpture produced by the Rumanian artistic counterculture.

I seem to notice that nearly all signs work like a KEEP LEFT sign. They move us around in space. ONE WAY. YIELD. MAKAWAO 2 MILES.

But the Dead Bomb Shelter sign doesn't move us around in space. It moves us in time.

It tells us a brief story. CAUTION: DEAD BOMB SHELTER, it says. It describes a former bomb shelter that once lay right under the concrete paving, right under your feet. The bomb-shelter hole got backfilled. Then the freshly-moved dirt did that dirty trick of settling. That's why the dip.

The sign transforms that obscure but particular spot from a glitch in the masonry to an archeological site. It reminds us to see and to live, even as we rush around town. It helps to compensate for the grievous loss of the community-building

Makawao dump.

It's a timely notice.

I wrote these essays to be timely notices, too.

These essays are not designed to travel efficiently through space. When they make a turn, it's generally a hairpin turn – just like the road that twists past my driveway here in the gulch country of this wave-bashed mountain I live on. Along the road you'll find the most harmonious mix of complete unlikeliness – here in this loose community of 17 cultures where cattle graze under coconut trees and breakfast might well turn out to be Spam musubi and a donut, chased by a small tub of wheat grass juice.

My neighbors manage to make good sense out of strange ingredients that life keeps handing them, and I'd be happy to have said that I did the same.

For the sake of this collection, let's just say that I learned my trade at the Makawao dump – where everything was honest and solid (though it was transforming before your very eyes from chattel to compost!). And everything was welcome, no matter how it arrived.

And in that mess a glorious work was accomplished, a community. And the community grew – not because of the artful piles of rubbish, but because of the universal kindness that sits like a secret pearl inside the crusty oyster of the human heart.

I'd be satisfied if these essays served as much use.

P.S. Over the brief time that's passed since I wrote the words above, the "Dead Bomb Shelter" sign has disappeared. Now they've got an efficient little drain in the former puddle, and no one will have to be inconvenienced by noticing. But for those of us who remember the "Dead Bomb Shelter" sign, – now THOSE were the good old days!....

THE PLACE

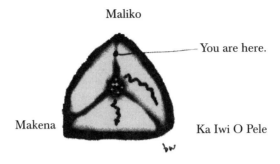

Maliko

You are here.

Makena

Ka Iwi O Pele

Makawao from 20,000 feet in the air

"It's all in how you see it!" says geologist Earl Onaga as we rise straight into the sky above the Makawao crossroads.

"Most of the time, people only get the close-up view of things – buildings, streets, other people. With this Sky-Hoist, though, we'll get the MACRO view. We'll REALLY be able to see where you Upcountry folks live."

"How high up are we going?" I say.

You have to watch what you ask for. When I asked Earl to show me the physical geography of Makawao, I should have specified a WALKING tour. The air's getting colder already, and I'm gripping the rim of the little two-person bucket that's lifting us into outer space.

I hate heights.

"About 20,000 feet," says Earl calmly. "About twice as high as the summit of Haleakala Crater."

"Swell."

We're rising at a dizzying speed, and my ears are popping like champagne corks at an inaugural ball. The towns and roads below are disappearing, and the patterns of trees and fields take over. Now Makawao is little more than a dark green cross formed by treetops. I see rumpled, golden-green pastures. Designer-drawn, almost violet pineapple fields. Thick dark fur-patches of forest.

Earl's happy. "Not a cloud! What a day!" he says. "Now, look for the BIG PATTERNS."

"Looks pretty random to me."

"That's 'cause we're not high enough. Gotta go WAY up."

"Swell."

By the time we finally stop, the sky is purple. East Maui looks about the size of a turkey platter. My knees are seismic.

"Excellent," says Earl. "Now you'll see. Ignore West Maui; that's a separate mountain. Focus on Haleakala, and tell me—what shape is it?"

"Kinda round."

"No."

I look again, then I see it.

"A triangle."

"Yes. Actually, Haleakala is a 3-sided pyramid. Three faces, with three separate, long ridges radiating out from the crater to the sea. See 'em? They're called RIFTS – long torn places where lava boiled out whenever the volcano was active."

"I can see lots of little round hills along the rifts."

"Pu'us. Cinder cones. Volcanic activity along the rifts, that's why."

We look at the rifts one by one. The Southwest Rift runs from the summit through Polipoli Forest, right down the middle of 'Ulupalakua Ranch, then ends at Makena. From there, we look eastward across the long, softly wavy flank, past Kanaio and Kahikinui, past where the even face is gouged by Kaupo Gap, then we see the East Ridge. It runs from the Paliku-Cabin end of the crater straight to Hana.

"Not quite to Hana," corrects Earl. "I'd put Hana Bay to the north of it, and 'Ohe'o – you know, Seven Pools – to the south.

I'd say the rift ends at Ka Iwi O Pele, that pu'u next to Koki Beach. Now run your eyes along the Hana Road flank of the pyramid. There's Ko'olau Gap."

"How come those gaps are there, anyway?"

"The bowl filled with water and overflowed, and washed a couple of cracks. Now, look where YOU live."

The North Rift. Down through Olinda, Makawao, Ha'iku, ending at Maliko Bay and Pauwela Point.

"We live on a pyramid edge!"

"Yep. Baldwin Avenue pretty much runs along the rift-line. You know," he adds, "that road used to be the way to get to the crater. When Mark Twain came here over a hundred years ago, he took that route to the summit."

"The North Rift. That's why our area has so many pu'us."

"That's right. There's Pu'u O Umi, above Maliko Bay. There's that beautiful pu'u on Kauhikoa Road, another one on Lower 'Ulumalu, where people have just started building houses. And there's Giggle Hill. Now look at all three pyramid faces. How are they different?"

"The one between the North Ridge and the East Ridge, the Hana Road part, it's all covered with trees. It's all full of gullies and ridges."

"Right. It faces directly into the trade winds. When you live in Makawao, you're not only on the North Ridge, but you're also right where the trade winds break. Right over your head. That's why it's called Ma-ka-wao. 'START-OF-THE-JUNGLE.'"

"Oh."

"Actually, the word 'wao' means any kind of wilderness or uninhabited region – the abode of gods, spirits, and ghosts."

"Wow," I say. "Wao."

"You know what a wilderness is?" says Earl.

"Wao," I say again. I peek through my fingers and see a jet airplane cruising along, far below me. I'm keeping my comments short. Anything to keep from whimpering. "Wow," I say.

"A wilderness is anything that 'wilders.' And if you live near the wilderness, most of the time you're pretty much 'bewildered.' Get it?"

"Uh huh. Bewildered. Got it."

"That's why you people are all crazy. You live on a knife-edge where the land exploded for a million years. On the left side, where it's dry, it's cactus and curbs and clear skies. On the right, people raise tilapia fish in their driveways and swing from the trees. I wouldn't expect a high degree of social organization."

"But we can get along, don't you think?"

He smiles. "Any other questions?"

"Just one. How fast does this bucket drop?"

"Hold on," he says.

Witness reports leaping dog, other flying beasts

I quit smoking cigarettes. It's been over a week, and I feel great. I could bite a piece of re-bar in half. I could arm-wrestle a backhoe. My brain's getting so much oxygen that it can't even think straight. I haven't written a paragraph in a week. Just short sentences. Very. Disconnected.

You know how it is when you blow up a balloon and pinch the end and then hold it over your head and let it go? My brain. My brain on oxygen.

So THIS is what it feels like, to be like all you non-smokers. Honestly, how can you stand it? Too much oxygen is a danger-ous thing. It turns breathing into a martial art, an aikido thing. One good lung-full and you're ready, just in case you need to leap into the air and kick the back of someone's head. World peace is obviously out of the question, here in this aerobic world where no peace pipes are passed. Peace may be out of the ques-tion, but I'm telling you one thing:

Nothing's gonna upset me.

I'm under control. Willpower. Nothing's gonna upset me, not

even the fact that my dog's legs are too short.

In fact, the main problem I have experienced in researching this essay is the embarrassing stumpiness of my dog's legs. Plus the excess oxygen that's rattling my brain. Plus the ever-present risk that this essay will turn out to be truly pointless. Plus the chronic spinelessness of American public opinion and the near-impossibility of finding true love in an increasingly fragmented, expanding universe.

Excuse me while I chew on this re-bar for a minute.

Knowing that my thought process is going to be impaired this week, I decide to let my dog, Makapuʻu, write the essay instead. I decide to drive him to Makawao, then follow him around while he points out the sights and smells that most interest him. Let HIM do all the sustained thinking for a change.

Good plan, but for one flaw.

My dog can't jump into my truck anymore. Don't laugh. This is a serious matter when you live Upcountry.

My old truck – now there was a jump he could make! He could FLY in there, like a thick-chested wolf leaping an ice-choked gorge to bring meat back to the brush-masked cave. To the future! To the rescue! Hound, leaping! Man, smoking! Ah those were the days.

My new truck is a 4 X 4; the tailgate's higher than the old one's used to be. That's the problem. To tell the whole truth, my dog's not as svelte as he used to be. That's the other part of the problem. In fact, he's not even as svelte as my old TRUCK used to be!

Picture a saddle thrown over a piano bench and you'll get a pretty good sense of my dog's dimensions. Evolution has not selected him as one of its soaring, leaping creatures. Even when he used to get into the old truck, he always looked so serious about it that you knew he was bluffing. You knew he was scared.

The first time I ever called him to jump into my new truck, when he tried to jump but only his front paws made it, and then when he fell, clawing away at the tailgate, that was the first time

I ever realized that a dog can feel humiliated. He just walked away. That was that. He'd made a complete fool of himself, he was perfectly willing to admit it to anyone, but he wasn't going to hang around to find out who cared. He certainly wasn't going to fall on his doggie ass, his stiff little legs exposed and wiggling in the air, while attempting to jump that high ever again.

After that, I had to pick him up, all 93 pounds of hair and grease and Alpo, to get him into the new truck. Usually now I'll back the truck up to a grassy slope next to my driveway. What I need is a mutt-sized cattle chute.

Despite the hassle, I do like to take the dog out into the community. If you own a truck, you know why. Once we get rolling, Makapu'u goes wild with joy. He sticks his snout into the wind and sucks up, yawns up, all the smelly news of Maui and of its people and of its many cultures of dogs. His ears flap back and forth like car wash soap slappers. His tiny round dome of a skull and the big goopy grin indicate that all his information is pretty simple and tidy.

Just what I need for this no-nicotine essay. Something that makes simple sense.

So the dog and I park on Baldwin Avenue down by Nakui Street, across from David Warren's art studio. I drop the tailgate. The dog looks over the edge, then sits down again. He's not going to jump out. After all, how's he gonna get back in again?

"Come on," I say. "Stop worrying. I've got an article to write."

The fool trusts me, and jumps. He hits the ground running, and he goes right for the most interesting spot in the whole town of Makawao – which is a little row of croton bushes jutting out from the front door of that little house on the corner of Nakui.

Underneath those bushes, my dog finds 10,000 smells; he stays under there, sniffing, for at least 15 minutes. I imagine that he's discovered the entire history of Makawao, recorded in a kind of museum of smell-messages that were left by and for dogs. I've never really noticed those bushes before, but they are (for dogs, anyway) the be-all and the end-all.

When Makapuʻu comes out from under those bushes, he's ready to go home. He's smelled it all.

"Oh no," I insist. "We're going to tour this town. Now get walking!"

Kris Dixon, the Makawao Community Police Officer, comes by. Her office is in that little house where the bushes are full of information. We chat. She asks how old the dog is.

"Five or six," I say. I realize that I don't know my dog's age because I never celebrate my dog's birthday. I realize for the first time how much I hate the whole tradition of counting birthdays. I'm sorry I know how old I am, and I don't want any of you counting up how many years I've wasted when my birthday comes around next time. Remember that. I'm a reformed smoker. I'm alive, that's all. I don't need to keep score.

"Five or six? Is that all?" says Officer Dixon. "Looks like he needs to jog a little bit."

Because Officer Dixon is a slender and well-meaning woman, the dog and I decide not to strike up a debate on the issue. Instead, he takes me on a short tour of Makawao. Very short. From the dog's point of view, the whole town can be summarized in the following sentences:

• The grass in front of Silversword Stoves is full of interesting messages; sniff there.

   • A plastic bin that once held dried octopus legs is lying on the sidewalk, crushed; this is definitely the most exciting object in the entire town.

   • You'll want to cross the street so that you can walk your nose right past Rodeo Store's deli counter. Then you'll want to cross back so that you can walk your nose past Komodas.

   • You can lie in the shade in front of Crossroads Caffe, on the corner, and protect the whole town from traffic accidents.

That's the tour. Not very thrilling for a grouchy ex-smoker, but thrilling enough for a dog. When I call, "Let's go!" he runs back down the street, trying to leap into every car and truck in town.

When I drop the tailgate of my truck and turn around to hoist him up (somehow), he is already in the air! He's sailing past my ear in a golden blur!

He's leaping, just like a lawn mower that's trying to set a pole-vaulting record. His rear paws hit the top edge of the tailgate, and I grab the fur around his tail and boost him into the bed of the truck. The look on his face says this:

"See? It's attitude!"

Explosive leaps. Eruptions of oxygen. Flying through space in a burst of inadequate legs. This whole town, all of Upcountry Maui, is re-created every day by all of us as we stumble forth with our attitudes. I disagree with every one of you! And yet look at what we all manage to agree on, every day, as if we know what we mean when we say "Makawao."

I look up, and there are dogs flying everywhere – terriers, poi dogs, pit bulls, Chihuahuas, Great Danes, sailing over the store tops and the trees. Soon Holsteins and Aberdeen Angus cows are soaring through the sky, and above them appaloosas and palominos. Peace may be out of the question, but happiness on a volcanic island gets doled out in unforgettable bursts.

Doing our jobs in the big rain

A thousand kinds of rain come down on the Haʻiku side. They generally sweep in from Hana, billow up to Olinda, splash over Makawao, then break apart into the dry air as they blow toward Pukalani.

Of these, there is one kind that everyone knows – that big, big.... If it kept up for two days, it would wash all of us, and all of our artifacts, right off the face of the mountain. That's the kind I'm talking about.

I love that kind of rain.

I'm not stupid enough to think it's safe, or fun. That rain once killed a friend of mine. I've seen it destroy cars. For three days once I fought against it to save my house, and then only partially succeeded.

After that, my sons and some friends and I built a rock wall, a tough, gracefully curved stone shoulder thrown against any flash floods. It runs 100 feet and stands higher than our heads where it brunts against a flood, sweeping left with a bullfighter move to fool the water past the house into a deeper gulch.

Only a handful of us can remember the re-bar and beer cans and sweat that we dropped into the wall and buried forever into mortar and rubble. Over the past four years, the wall has taken on a tawny greenish cast. Ha'iku has accepted it.

Now I look at this wall with an Egyptian satisfaction. This rock monument will outlast me, and outlast my wooden house. I think that it might last thousands of years; other humans will live near this wall and wonder about its builders. Even if humans disappear, it will still do what it does.

Its bow perfectly counters the water's bow, and when rock and water slide together in these big rains that I'm talking about, one holding the line and the other testing it, I don't see competition so much as a perfect agreement.

The wall grew out of an agreement that the big rain demanded.

When it's raining seriously at dawn, you know you're in for a day of such agreements. The cold rain slaps against everything, pushing against the branches so that they twist and turn. The dog keeps pacing and shifting on the deck, then drops loudly, his snout pushed into the weather, his eyes cocking back and forth. Dawn comes slow and approximate in one of those rattling gray skies.

By ten o'clock, all heaven has broken loose. Wet drumming shakes the roof. It says: if the water can't do it, then the crackling and pounding itself intends to drown us out, drown out all of our protected activities. Liquid crystal comes sheeting off the roof, as if we'd built the place under a waterfall.

And then, unbelievably, the percussion-chaos gets even louder. People stop what they're doing, just stop. And then it gets even louder.

The roads can never hold it all. If you live on this side, you know where the bad places will be, the temporary riverbeds and short-term ponds where you need to drive.

Each storm will dump with a different intensity on different roads. In one storm, Upper 'Ulumalu will heave a gorge-full of dirt down into a swamped 5-Corners intersection; in another, a whole lake will cut you off from Hanzawa Store. Another time, Peahi will flood, or Kokomo Road will turn into a miles-long waterslide, perfect for hydroplaning into a catastrophe.

These roads are not roads, not any longer, not when the big rain hits. They reveal themselves to be sluices, sluices we built to hasten the destruction of this single mountain we live on, Haleakala. The pine roads, soaked to a state of truck-swallowing mush, disgorge yards and yards of fresh red earth. The new homes, too, give up some of their costly acreage every time it hits like this. I always see tons of Upcountry land heading to sea when our roads turn into these sluices.

In the big picture, that's what we're doing here. We think we are building, but we're doing the opposite – eroding, upsetting, gouging loose the earth, doing the same damage as pigs, only more. No matter what we build, we're doing the water's work.

Whenever I see that rich red current coursing along the roads, clogging the culverts, carrying tree parts and hubcaps, empty vodka bottles, shoes, dead chickens, but mostly earth, earth, earth, I can see it: UPCOUNTRY IS GOING DOWN.

Don't worry, though. This is not just erosion. This is inevitable. Our pig-work just hastens the inevitable. Now that the volcano has quit (supposedly), it's only a matter of time till Haleakala gets beaten back into the sea. The mountain is inchly fleeing northward, all the while chased and beaten and savagely beaten by kai and wai, that is by salt water and fresh water, sinking under its own weight and crumbling apart until that far day when it will finally dwindle into a sand shoal, or an atoll, or a rock outcropping for seabirds to mass on, fat seals to haul their fertile bodies onto.

We're here to help that happen.

Perhaps this is why my neighbors and I are always in a good mood, an excited state of friendliness, whenever the big rain comes down. Every guy with a backhoe is out on the road in a yellow slicker, big pinwheels of water spraying off his back tires. The linemen for the electric company go to work in the worst of it; the county road crews do heroic deeds in the downpours. I never resent my utility bills or my taxes during the big rain. On those days, anyone who moves meets some kind of adventure. Getting into a store safely is an achievement, a shared achievement, and so is getting home again. We share a danger, but it's a danger we can manage (as long as we work together), a danger with its quiet purpose of pushing forward the water's battle, a danger that frees us from the lonely and anxious feeling that we're in charge, somehow, of the whole mess – we, with our little bills and businesses and tightly-held beliefs.

After all, you can hold water for a brief time, and you can fool it into going left or right, but you can never control the stuff. Not only that, you can never really get upset with water. Despite its destructive force, water is entirely simple and innocent. It's a collective system of pure logic, triggered by one and only one desire: DOWNWARD. Any means to that end.

We can catch it, freeze it, drink it, walk it around inside our bodies, flush it, fight it, carry it, ride it, wipe it up, and drown in it – but in the end, we're all doing water's job. We're all in agreement with its plan to conquer the bony, inhospitable earth.

Despite all our beautiful, liquid thoughts to the contrary, we're really no more than two-legged sacks of organized water stalking forth to get the job done – expendable, highly specialized advance troops built to take the heat of a resentful sun.

Then, when the big rain finally settles back at the end of a turbulent, truly Ha'iku day, you almost have to laugh. This has been quite a visit. You step out into the yard. The clouds are breaking up, and some iron-hard stars are piercing through the black gaps.

You hear a distant gurgling in the hills and the gulches. The wind stirs around, and five fresh drops of the stuff fly off a banana leaf and hit you on the face. You and the land you live on. Once again, you've made the agreement.

A Solution to Makawao's Parking Problem

At sunset, you can park your old buggy in Makawao without much trouble. Most everyone else has gone home – eating, or getting ready to eat, or just plain hiding out.

The sky turns thick with color then, mostly lavenders backed up with a strange orange. A car will go past maybe once a minute. After its engine rips the air and passes, though, you get the weird sensation of actually noticing the town itself.

For once, you hear electricity buzzing in the power poles, up at the top where they're clotted with black cables stretching every which way, like bicycle spokes. All the trees speak up, rattling behind the funky shops in the gathering winds. The slam of a car door sounds four times louder than it does at noon.

The slanty parking slots in front of Rodeo Store, on the Ha'iku side of Baldwin Avenue and up close to the stop sign, those are filled. The parking places parallel to the sidewalk on the other side, from Makawao Steak House up to Silversword Stoves – those are all taken. Other than that, you've got lots of choices.

That's the way our little town should be, I guess. Not much happening.

At mid-day, this is a whole different place. Now you've got TRAFFIC. Rams. Rangers. Broncos. Blazers. Tow trucks. Here comes Earl Calasa, banging through the intersection in his banged-up salty-red hauler, one of the hardest-working trucks on the mountain. An MEO bus turns the corner with a full load of aunties and tutus. White trucks roar out of the county baseyard, king cabs with six big men and their shovels.

You have to shout above it all. Above the whining of loose belts and the high metal whistling of worn brakes. Above the deep tuba roars of gunned engine guts. Above the scratch and bang of tires smearing the gravel and bouncing on the drain covers. Then it stops for a moment. Silence drops like a hundred dollar bill. A single mynah gets his chance and takes it.

Chip. Chip. Chip.

But even in that silence, you hear the overall murmur of engines, like a sound track in a movie when you don't know why but you know something bad's about to happen. Suddenly, a hot-looking wahine in black shades and a black Datsun with black-tinted windows peels around the corner, her pounding reggae building up from the right then sinking away to your left.

Suddenly, 200 cars are all in a knot. People are backing out where they can't see. Drivers are slaloming around a big parked LeSabre that just couldn't pull in far enough, no matter what. A rusty panel truck, built like a Matson container, same thing – taking up half the roadway. The Waterman flatbed is delivering, and all of his water jugs sparkle like plastic blue ice. He's blocking the fire hydrant. But he's got no choice.

Jaywalkers cross wherever they can; they go, cars stop, they stop, they go, cars go. It's a dance. Then a herd of downhill bikers sails through, all in their poolball-green helmets, nervously squeezing their handbrakes with all the grim determination of somebody trying to gaff a shark in knee-high water. Their leader, riding no-handed, is turned around in his seat and shouting like a sailor, KEEP IN LINE! DON'T LOOK BACK! ONE FALSE MOVE AND YOU'RE DEAD!

Some people have called the town "dysfunctional" on account of times like this, but I disagree. Or maybe I just like dysfunctional towns. Because I've seen "functional" towns, and I'll tell you what.

Functional sucks.

Say "functional," and I think of certain towns I've visited in Orange County, California, where any house is painted one of three legislated color combinations and you get a fine if you leave your garage door open longer than 20 minutes. In a town like that, they've got sidewalks wider than Baldwin Avenue — on both sides of the street. And no one's on those sidewalks.

Everyone's driving. They're driving with windows rolled up on one of those eight extra-wide lanes that any "functional" town provides even when it has far less traffic than Makawao gets when St. Joseph's Church finishes High Mass.

To walk on those runway-sized sidewalks is to know a soul-killing loneliness. The only other pedestrian you see is way off in the distance, an old Mexican woman, someone's servant, pushing a shopping cart and hiding inside a dark, toothless silence.

You start to walk from one side of the street to the other, and a dread feeling strikes you halfway across that asphalt Sahara. Suppose your heart gives out! Suppose you sprawl flat across one of those mirage-wet lanes, crying out with a death-shriek! Your final glance would take in the grillwork of an approaching car. Its turn indicator would click on. The car would move into some other extra-functional lane, leaving you and your dysfunctional behavior to the disposal of well-paid municipal authorities.

If it's a parking place you want, now there's the place to get one. If you chopped the Makawao strip into portable pieces, shipped them all to Orange County, and spread them out over one of those mega-boulevards, the whole town would simply disappear.

I count 85 parking spots on Makawao Avenue, from the 3-way stop sign (the very heart of confusion) to the end of the commercial strip down by the Steak House. This includes the Komoda's lot, which is (wink wink) just for the Komodas. In that stretch we have about 30 businesses.

And how many cars go through town every day? I'm sure someone's got the official count, but who cares. Suppose we figure one car every five seconds for the 12 busiest traffic hours of the day. That's 8,640. Add a bit more for the other 12 hours – call it 10,000 a day.

What a beautiful, big figure! What a town! What a miracle!

Suppose that one day, maybe today, everyone who's driving through town needs to stop and park. Now picture that – almost 120 cars for every parking spot. Picture cars piled on cars nearly 600 feet high, higher than any high-rise tower in Honolulu. If that ever happens, I hope to heaven that I'll be there.

In fact, I will be there. After all, who are those 10,000 people?

Us. The most diverse group of 10,000 you could assemble anywhere on this planet. Pig farmers and preachers, plumbers, pizza-makers, punks, and pineapple pickers. Cowpokes and cruisers, clerks, accountants, and clothes merchants. Not to mention the alarming mix of races, languages, creeds, ages, cares, histories. You know what I'm talking about.

Makawao makes us mix. Unlike many other towns, it serves this special purpose. Starting with the 3-way stop, where we have to halt, halt again, wave at each other, guess what each other will do, cuss under our breaths, thank each other, the whole trip through town is an exercise in community interaction. Every trip makes us test our prejudices and look each other in the face.

If Baldwin Avenue was a stream-lined, multi-lane thoroughfare, would we ever do that: look each other in the face? If we could zip through town, would we be a better community?

Go ahead and laugh, if you like, but here's my truth. I like the inconvenience.

I like that we all have to take care of each other while we back in and out of broken driveways, remember how to parallel park while eight waiting drivers make wisecracks, bend the law while we jaywalk – and meanwhile, don't forget, we're all taking care of that guy's extra-long LeSabre.

I'm telling you my solution to the parking problem. Take it. Take it as an exercise in community fitness.

If all of us did (and most of us do), we'd be in heaven. Because I guess that heaven is a loud, disorganized, and – above all – wonderfully dysfunctional place.

my town, its parade, its parade, and its parade

At the appointed time and day, people in my community go to the town's busiest street and, standing or sitting, block up the sidewalks.

They wear clothing that they wouldn't normally wear in public – for example, a cowboy hat that sits on the high shelf in the closet every other day of the year.

This year a man tied the string of a helium balloon to the adjustment strap on the back of his baseball cap. I don't believe this man would do such a thing on any normal day – stand around on the street with a balloon floating over his head.

(But you know, I can't be sure of that. In my town, people will wear turbans, lava-lavas, chaps, string bikinis, live animals, aura-sensitive crystal tiaras, hip boots, glitter – even balloons, both partly and fully inflated – on any given day of the week.)

On this appointed day, as I was saying, some people clump on the sidewalk while other people walk or ride slowly along the middle of the street so that they can be looked at.

This is called a parade.

The distinction between the people who do nothing on the sidewalks and the people who pass in front of them is so important that a bright yellow plastic tape marks the symbolic border between them. Black letters in the tape spell, repeatedly, "Crime Scene Do Not Pass."

The purpose of a parade is to give lots of people the chance to look at other people without much of a chance that they'll look back. We humans love to do that.

(What else are the movies all about, then, if you don't really think so?)

If you're willing to take the walk, people will spend a whole morning standing on a public street wearing a balloon just to have the chance to look at you when you do that.

At least, in my town on the 4th of July that's what we like to do.

We also like to look at horses. (In some cases, we prefer to look at the horses.)

We on the sidewalks all have one reason to be there, and one alone – to stare impolitely from behind sunglasses and say anything we want without caring who hears. The rest of the year we keep our eye contact to quick glances and keep our thoughts to ourselves, but this is a holiday. On holidays, social order breaks down; that's why we have holidays.

On the holiday called Independence Day, we get to look until our appetites are crammed. Such pleasure does not make us independent, but it does make us feel free. Liberated.

According to a recent Gallup poll, 72 percent of Americans agree that, in a democracy, personal freedom is more important than equality. In my town, we take the personal freedom to stare and gawk at each other on July 4th, and some of us drink beer a little earlier in the day than usual, and that's fun.

But here's the interesting question. Why do people volunteer to *march* in a parade, to pass between these eyeball firing squads? Why do they want to move through the main artery of the town, like some sort of vital community blood?

They have reasons. These reasons are many and complicated.

This year I noticed 3 – as if I were watching 3 parades pass at once, each intermingled with the other.

The first reason would seem to be the national joy of patriotism, because the color guard comes early in the parade, borne on a black mare that prances and back-steps toward the crowd. The galvanized roofs of the town's main shops – whose wooden walls have cliffed against the tropical weather for so long that their hides have turned the texture of old leather – wear a mile-long hat band of Old Glory pennants. Everywhere we look the U.S. flag snaps like big sparks off a car battery. Electrifying. Incapable of rest.

Because it's the theme of the parade, I keep thinking about the high ideal of independence. You'd think an island in the Pacific would be as independent as it gets. And it sure is. Until you run out of toilet paper – which we did back in the early 70s. But the barges and planes have been more reliable since.

We did manage to liberate one of the islands in our county from a hostile government that dropped tons of bombs on the place and shattered its fragile ecosystem. But now it'll take billions to clean up the mess, and the hostile government refuses to pay the bill because times are tough.

And that hostile government is us.

Like lots of Americans, I was born wishing for a bomb shelter and now I have a piece of the Berlin Wall sitting on my desk. I've been through hurricanes and earthquakes; I like harvesting bananas, or nearly anything. I am an ordinary man.

And I think that Dependence deserves its day.

As usual on July 4th, I'm thinking too much. Forgetting the whole point. I take a lesson from my neighbor, who says to me after the color guard passes – in his voice thick with Scottish snare-drum rattlings – "Not one person took off the hat when the colors walked by. Except for an alien. Me."

He looks at my cowboy hat, which is on my head, and says, "When you come here next year, please take notice of how many f–ing guys take off their hats when the flag goes by. It's something I've observed for 28 years and I've only been a f–ing citizen since '81."

The national park rangers are hiking past now with brown ponies and a fine buckskin mule, the mule a rarity in these parts.

And then I begin to notice the 2nd obvious reason people dare to parade – for the personal joy of commerce. Commerce clearly dominates our little parade. Nearly everyone but the color guard is advertising a product or service.

The staff of the physical therapy clinic lets us admire the straightness of their spines while they show us a sign that reads "We Accept All Insurance." A concrete-pumping truck rolls past. "Pumping With Confidence." The Maui Stunt Men pass by on a flatbed, pretending to beat each other silly.

Every July 4th parade should feature this kind of shameless advertising, a great American tradition. Plus, it serves an important purpose where we live. Maui's merchants and entrepreneurs are gradually undermining the plantation economy that's kept my state in undemocratic, feudal bondage for 150 years.

But none of this has to do with independence. These people want us to need their well-massaged tendons, their well-pumped grout, and their well-faked disasters. They want us to depend on them.

In a truly independent community, would anyone at all show up for a parade?

Suddenly, a limousine service drives one of its gleaming white cars through the ogling throngs. Draped over the car, hood trunk and bumper, six good-looking women wear nothing but tiny Star-and-Stripes bikinis.

My neighbor starts in again. "And there's another thing. You should never wear the f–ing flag! Not even if... not that I...." But his voice trails off because he's concentrating so hard on the many images of Old Glory.

And then right behind the bikinis steps the Salvation Army,

ranks of somber young women, mostly Filipina, marching in derbies and straight, past-the-knee skirts.

The Parade Marshals have a sense of humor.

I notice the Parade Marshals now, sitting with dignity on their accommodating horses. Suddenly the rest of the parade looks a little frivolous.

After all, this is their parade, these men and women on horseback. They and their people have siphoned down and up from their families' ranches and gulches, and they're walking the gauntlet with grace and dignity, adults among children, heading for the rodeo grounds one mile up the hill.

They've replaced the police today, and they're governing the town from horseback. They aren't kidding. They're not selling anything, and I don't believe they're thinking much about the Republican agenda on Capitol Hill, nor about documents signed 220 years ago by somebody else's grandfather.

If I can guess their reason, a 3rd reason, for accepting the curious stares of all, it's this:

They come to reclaim the town.

They are the conscience of the land made visible; they are the rooted people. The affairs of town can't possibly rattle them. Double the number of shops? Tear them all down? These questions can't possibly strike at the heart of their experience of community.

Roots don't grow under shop roofs. They grow in soil mulched by the bodies of all who have gone before, pressed flat by hoofs and strong feet, watered with perspiration.

Our parade ends with street-sweeping trucks wire-whisking the roadway, stirring up a perfume of horse dung, asphalt, hot leather, crushed leaves. The machines are chased by a dragonfly that bobs up into a wide sky, a sky that's as blue and confident as a freshly washed razor.

This parade, I realize, has nothing to do with independence.

ⓑ

The tale of the brand-new building inspector

Once upon a recent time, an earnest young man came to Maui from Seattle, Washington. He just wanted to be free, live simply, have a good job, swim in the sea. He was tired of city life with all of its rules and controls.

In Seattle, he had worked as a building inspector. Maui, he could see, had many buildings that deserved inspection. Life on Maui would work more smoothly, he could tell, with more careful application of the rules and controls.

He had the madness of a newcomer. He wanted to make this place more like the place he'd fled.

He thought of himself as a missionary. He carried a rule book, just like the first missionaries. The missionaries' rule book had convinced the people of Maui to hide their behavior behind closed doors. The inspector's rule book specified exactly which kinds of doors to hide behind.

So the young man landed a job inspecting buildings for the County of Maui. For his first assignment, the chap was assigned to the under-inspected crossroads town of Makapiapia.

As he drove into Makapiapia, he could see the town for what it was. He didn't even have to get out of his truck for that. He could see that Makapiapia was a living testimony to the enduring power of corrugated tin roofing.

He was not fooled by the Western-style cut-out facades on the front of each store. He started looking past the High-Noon porches pasted to the dry plywood fronts of all the shops.

He was not charmed by the fresh paint on the few shops that had slapped it on, like old ladies who had smeared on bright lipstick even though they could no longer find the edges of their lips.

He saw that if you put a marble on the floor near the cash register of the general store, the marble would roll spontaneously down the aisle between the saimin packages and the sexy magazines, turn left at the taro chips, and then, just in front of the limp produce section, drop through a gap in the floor down to the bare dirt crawl space under the building where an ownerless Weimaraner slept every night.

In every board he saw dry rot and damp rot and fungus condominiums, the powdering corruptions of Time. He saw the mineral clogging of galvanized pipes, and he heard the rattling of inadequate roofing.

He saw high-voltage electrical wiring sheathed in what looked to him like peanut husks. He peeled away wallboard to find studs at 4-foot intervals, more or less. He witnessed the industry of termites; he grew familiar with their terrible dungpiles. He asked to see the Certificates of Occupancy of 63 shopkeepers.

Only two had them.

He saw that 82,976 people a day stomped through these shuddering shacks, 82,976 dreamers and fools and philosophers, loud-voiced sensualists, bearded mystics, pig farmers, and calloused survivors, none of whom gave the whispiest damn about the terrible dungpiles.

In fact, they loved the terrible dungpiles that pointed

upwards, in their tiny way, toward a human heaven.

As the wind tossed itself about the shops, and the rains coiled in and out, and the sun poured itself promiscuously anywhere, the good citizens of Makapiapia scarcely even heard the chorus of suitable whisperings that arose from all those terrible dung-piles – just so many more syllables in Time's long and appropriate language.

So the building inspector from Seattle announced that he was shutting down the entire town of Makapiapia.

That night, the merchants of Makapiapia met in a state of controlled panic, which was the only way they could ever meet. They gathered in the office of Larry Broadhurst, the chiropractor who kept a dagger strapped to his shin at all times.

There was the owner of a Chinese herbal medicine and crystal shop, three women who each imported Balinese demon masks and fake ikat fannypacks, a gelato merchant, a naturopath, and a sand-play therapist. Two oil painters and a seaweed sculptor came because they had studios in the little town. There was also the epileptic owner of a small locksmith shop and two restaurateurs – who had schemed in the car on the way over about setting up a meat boutique in the window facing the Ginseng Elixir Fountain. Leonard Breath, the colonic irrigationist who advertised "sterile disposable tips," he was there.

Not everyone came to the meeting. The florist was having a tonsillectomy. The town barber had only cussed at the building inspector, calling him a "stink haole troublemaker." That was the end of the issue for her. The long-time merchants, Japanese families, were having dinner in back of their stores; they didn't bother.

Taoana Tantra and Moondolphin, the lesbian owners of the Dust-To-Dust Maranatha Natural Food Store, had their regular prayer group to go to. A special guest was going to unveil evidence of reincarnation in the Bible. Since the philosphy of their relationship was "physical immortals do it forever," they felt the building inspector's problem was primarily a vibrational one, anyway. And the guy who owned the Booze Barn didn't come because he didn't give a damn.

The meeting lasted an hour and fifteen minutes. For an hour, everyone took turns saying the same thing: they were gonna stay open until somebody shut them down.

Someone suggested an organized appeal to the county. Leonard Breath, the colonic irrigationist, volunteered to spearhead the campaign. No one offered to join him, so the idea crapped out.

Then the meeting degenerated into a gripe session about vandalism. When Larry Broadhurst tried to demonstrate how to break a man's neck with a broom handle, most people went home.

The next day, Makapiapia opened quietly.

Shopkeepers scanned the street. They walked back and forth to each other's shops, then stood side-by-side, scanning.

"Nothing's going to happen," said one. "What could they do?" said the other.

"Nobody'd shut down a whole town!"

"Do you think?"

The gelato merchant put in a call to the governor's office, but then hung up when someone answered the phone.

In fact, nothing happened all day. Or ever. Except for this:

The building inspector from Seattle was quickly removed to a new position. He was placed in charge of a mobile unit dispatched by the county Animal Shelter.

He came back for the ownerless Weimaraner, but the citizens of Makapiapia drove him away. Later, he went into business for himself, offering a Home Buyers Inspection Service. Then his wife left him for a part-Hawaiian pot grower (also part owner of the Pono Pump Gym), who shot the tires off his pickup truck when he was chasing the renegade lovers through a cane field under a sickle moon.

After that, the building inspector moved back to Seattle.

ⓖ

THE PRICE
(YOU HAVE TO PAY)

Crime Watch:
the impossible does not come true

If it isn't easy, it's impossible.

- DUKE ELLINGTON

Most of the news I care about is summarized in the "Crime Watch" section of the local paper – little one-paragraph mentions of petty and unsolvable crimes that were reported to the Maui police. Let somebody else turn to the sports page, or drive up his blood pressure stewing over conditions in Haiti or North America or other islands.

Let somebody else study the comparables in the real estate classifieds, cussing under her breath. Give the comics to Junior; I can't understand them anymore.

I'd rather read about jimmied locks, rifled fannypacks, and hijacked roosters. When I brush against these stories, I feel most tormented by our common humanity, and most aware of the need to commit wholesome, safe, and relatively harmless crimes.

As a writer, I like "Crime Watch" because each paragraph tells a story about us. And so little of the story is told that I can freely imagine all the good parts – the why, the faces, the aftermath.

A woman in Kihei saw a man remove a screen and sneak into her kitchen. This was just after dawn. The man stole two weiners valued at 69 cents. He snuck away.

So it says in "Crime Watch."

Now, this interests me. Why the hot dogs? Why not the kim chee or the smoked octopus? Do weiners make the perfect breakfast food? Or was the thief a kind of poet, acting out the muffled sexiness of the personal violation called "breaking and entering?" Why not take ALL the weiners? And how much time, I wonder, did the police officer spend calculating the true market value of a single pair of weiners? And why did the woman who reported this incident watch, without intervening?

My mind races to fill in the details, but I must hold myself back. After all, both the weiner thief and the victim might be reading this article right now. My imagining has no right to cancel their fact.

In Kahului, a homeless woman left her purse in a phone booth. When she came back, all that she had – fifteen dollars – was gone.

I have been that down.

Once, when I was young and naive, I offered a man a ride in my old rusty Volkswagen bug, and that man pulled a knife on me, stealing everything I had. I think he got four dollars and seventy-three cents, mostly in coins. What I remember most of all is the shaking of my knees, because I wasn't used to the idea of getting carved up with a knife.

That wouldn't happen now. Not the knees. Not the Volkswagen. Not even the ride.

The two previously mentioned "Crime Watch" stories came from Kihei and Kahului. Normally, though, when I read "Crime Watch," I go right away to my own geographical area. I hate to admit this, but it's true; the further away the crime, the less I care. I always read "East Maui" and "Upcountry" first.

My neighborhood has its own big crimes. In fact, this statement is true of all neighborhoods: by its crimes shall you know it.

For instance, a Ha'iku man reported that his mailbox sustained $25 in damages "from an unknown instrument" – not, I assume, a clarinet. In a related story, a pasture gate right down the street from my house was struck by a car.

In my neighborhood, most of the big stories have to do with the breaking of inanimate objects.

In Ha'iku, people like to break things, especially things made of metal. Especially mailboxes, cars, guard rails. Especially after midnight, when Upcountry roads become insane bowling alleys, tires screaming and explosions of metal and glass. The happy, wild, loony nature of my neighbors makes itself obvious then. In the quiet night, I hear gleeful bursts of destruction, like fireworks – CRASH. KABLOOWEE. Wild laughter.

I understand this. Something inside of us just hates driving carefully all the time, paying car payments for five years, checking the oil, watching for little paint dings with their tell-tale streaks of rust. Most of us never once get the chance to drive the thing right into a wall at 80 miles an hour then stagger away from the wreck, shaken and drenched with sweat, fully alive, totally free, taking orders directly from God almighty himself.

For excitement, this kind of physical challenge must be second only to birth. I've seen such acts of daring take place many times, right in front of my house.

Too bad they cost so much.

Passionate spendthrifts, however, abound in my community, and the hubcaps, red glass, bent bumpers, and broken mirrors along the roadside where I live tell not so much of destruction as they tell of crazy yearning and the desire for transformation.

When I read my "Crime Watch," I look for the small but extravagant outbursts that characterize my people. Also, when I'm at my best, I sometimes remember to notice what's NOT there.

There are crimes that I never see in "Crime Watch."

My brother bought a house in Los Angeles several years ago. Now he and his wife have to explain to their children why they hear gunshots every night. I know a man who moved here from another part of that city only four months ago. He loved what he was doing over there. But he moved so that his son would be able to play in the front yard.

"I had a chain link fence and two hundred-pound dogs," he said. "It wasn't enough."

For the Chinese, this is the Year of the Dog. Citizens of Beijing, however, are not allowed to own dogs. In a park north of the city, citizens can rent a dog that they can walk. The price: 23 cents for ten minutes.

In April, Feng Quantang filed a lawsuit in Shenyang, China, asking for damages from the government because inspectors allegedly beat his illegal dog to death in front of him.

When I'm at my best, I remember some of the many crimes that we don't have to watch for.

India and Pakistan have been at war for the past nine years in a border dispute over the Siachen Glacier. No one can live on that glacier, yet the soldiers are shooting each other. For every soldier who gets shot, nine die from the blinding blizzards, the treacherous footing on ice-encrusted peaks, and wind-chilled temperatures of more than 150 degrees below zero.

No one from Ha'iku has volunteered to fight the noble battles of Siachen Glacier. This fact explains one of the many reasons I am happy to be here.

Mailboxes have it tough. For people, though – it's better than impossible.

Exquisite reasons for ordinary acts: driving

They say that the odds of an average person getting attacked by a shark are one in several million. The odds of getting hit by lightning on any given day are one in 250 million.

But these are not the statistics that changed Melvin Tanaka's life.

Melvin was sitting in his car waiting for his grandfather to come tottering out from Pukalani Superette with breakfast – six Spam musubi and two cans of Fanta. Somebody had left a copy of Reader's Digest in his car, so he was flipping through it and then he found this list of interesting statistics.

He found out that the odds of losing your virginity between the months of March and August are nearly one in 10. ("Did I...?" Melvin asked himself, but he couldn't remember.) And if you think you've seen a flying saucer, join 10 percent of Americans. ("Never did," thought Melvin. Being a practical kind of guy, he added, "And I never going see one, too.")

But none of these statistics would make a person want to drive with insane slowness.

Then he read the odds for dying in a car crash – one in 125. Car travel is 10 times more dangerous than flying and 25 times riskier than taking the bus.

(If there was a bus.)

Still, he didn't think too much about it. (That's the risk you take, he thought.)

But then he found out the fact. The terrible fact. Certain cars are more dangerous than others, said the article.

And it listed the high-risk cars. It listed all the cars that Melvin loves. Corvettes and Camaros. Firebirds and Fieros.

Folks who drive those-kind cars face a one in 30 chance of death in a crash.

He blinked and looked again. Yes, the chance that he, Melvin, could die in the crash of a Nissan 300ZX is one in 30.

One in 30!

("That's like one day out of a month," he thought. "That's like one day in every month some guy's going come jumping up from out of the bushes and start shooting, li' dat. AT ME.") Melvin felt as though someone had just hit him in the chest with a dead ahi.

Melvin Tanaka DRIVES a Nissan 300ZX.

Very slowly. Ever since that day.

Melvin pulled out of the Pook-Soop parking lot, thinking hard. He wondered if he would he would be alive enough to eat Spam musubi when he was 82 years old, like his grandfather. And then, crossing the Pukalani bypass, he almost got clipped on the back fender by a Volvo coming down from Kula. "Slow down," he shouted.

He drove to Makawao at 20 miles per hour. It felt good.

I'll tell you. Melvin Tanaka is one hard-headed guy. When he decides to drive slow, he drives very slow. He don't care about nobody else.

He and his charcoal-gray Nissan 300ZX will never exceed the speed limit. Not any more. "If it's a risk, it's a stupid risk" – that's Melvin's motto now.

And Melvin's not alone. When he snapped like that and made up his mind to "go the limit," he joined approximately 20

percent of the drivers who pass through the Upcountry town of
Makawao.

He has even gone so far as to write a letter to the editor of a
certain local newspaper. He even had a bumper sticker made,
that says this:

"Dare For Drive Slow."

You can spot Melvin everywhere he goes. He always has five
cars behind him, or seven, or nine. The cars are all nearly
touching bumpers. And they're all driving like Melvin: slow.

You can see the tight lips and the frowns on the drivers' faces;
you see lips moving, forming hostile words. Drivers lean their
heads out the window and stare, trying to concentrate so hard
that their stink-eye will turn into a laser death-ray and blow
Melvin's Nissan right off the road.

Behind him you can see a convertible Beamer, a rented
Tracker, then a backhoe. Even a backhoe is faster than Melvin
Tanaka.

After that comes a higher-consciousness Datsun, its rusty
parts held together with bumper stickers, road grime, and good
will. ("Miracles Happen!")

Then comes pounding a huge-tired, jewel-blue truck full of
large Polynesian men. You can hear them yelling back there.

And up in front Melvin is cruising. Got his dark shades on.
He's got his rear-view mirror cranked to the side so he doesn't
have to look behind. He's got plenty of time. He left the house
30 minutes early.

Melvin is the leader. He has formed a community.

Why don't they pass him, you ask? Why, you're obviously a
stranger to these regions. The rest of America may be scram-
bling to find an on-ramp to the digital world traffic jam, but our
rumpled district is filled with 2-lane, shoulderless strands of
asphalt spaghetti, some of them with hairpins so tight that you
can drop your cigar out the window at the top of the curve then
catch it again yourself as you're straightening out.

We have just about as much experience on four lane highways as we have with making snowmen.

In Upcountry Maui, you don't pass. You gather.

Here, you can't move out onto the street without having relationships of all kinds. The streets make us meet each other, and the rules of the road are deeply ingrained in the way we treat each other. And here is one of the most unbreakable rules of the road:

Every day, to one degree or another, the slowest person sets the pace.

Laugh if you want, but it seems to me that Melvin's chain gang of traffic, going down Kaupakalua Road like a bobsled team on slow replay, that this is a perfect symbol for our times. This is what it means to live in a democracy.

In a democracy, all of us are equal. All of us are equally slow.

The leaders get in front because everyone else is too swift to bother with the job. The leaders are always too cautious or too incompetent to keep up with the pace and too selfish to pull over and get out of the way.

The swift, of course, have it bad in a democracy. People with fire in their blood are always stuck in the back, frustrated, angry. And most people are pressed in the middle, feeling pressure from both front and back. Checking their watches.

It's democracy, I tell you, same as in Washington, D.C. In front we have our leaders – Jesse Helms, for example, is head of the Senate Foreign Relations Committee. In the rear, we see America's city skies, punctuated with gunfire. The rest of us, here in the middle, we have newspapers and pharmaceuticals.

The only question is: how do you feel about your place in the rhumba line?

Melvin liked his.

After six months of slowness, he was starting to get a swelled head. He liked being in charge, setting the pace for everyone. His friends got mad at him. "Brah," they said, "the speed limit means don't go SLOWER than that!" He ignored them.

Then, one day, it happened. He was coming around a curve with a dozen cars behind when, suddenly, he had to step on the brake. Someone was in front of him!

In a white Nissan 300ZX. Going twice as slow! When the car went around curves, the driver put on her blinkers.

She was pretty, she was young, and she was singing as she drove.

Melvin got one good look at her (on a hairpin turn), and his heart started to pound. A blowhole of love geysered in his chest. When, after a mile or so, she pulled off the road to visit with a newly born foal in a thick green pasture, Melvin pulled over, too.

The traffic whizzed by. Few people noticed the two strangers, hands on the fence standing side by side looking at the baby horse, a rainbow arching over the pasture.

No one knows what the odds are for falling in love while driving a Nissan 300ZX. But at this time of year, the odds of seeing a rainbow on Kaupakalua Road on any given day are the best there can be.

One in one.

If you can't take this one, fine. I don't wanna know.

I'm forcing myself to write this. I can barely squeeze the words out. My shoulders are bunched up so tight I feel as if my neck is one big turnbuckle twisting tighter and tighter, and I keep panting and muttering, and every once in a while I jump out of my chair to go somewhere but there's nowhere to go, and my editor Carla's going to kill me if I don't get this thing done.

The problem is my topic. Stay with me now. I guarantee you'll be STRUCK with the desire to stop reading as soon as I tell you. But don't you dare.

I'm writing about re...

re... re... re...

That re... thing.

You know, that thing where you take all that rubbish and all that poopoo kind stuff and instead of just throwing it out shazam like you're the king of the universe or something, instead of that, you take each piece and look at it again and wash it off or peel off the label and put it in little bags or boxes, all sorted out like you're saving it all for some kind of weird museum, the family poop museum.

RECYCLING.

I'll tell you right now. I don't want to write about it, and I don't want to do it. "Don't play with your poopoo!" That's what my dad taught me.

My dad also taught me that bow ties are cool, that Walt Disney makes the only movies worth watching, and that I'd be handicapped all my life if I didn't know how to use a slide rule.

Dad was right. Then. I'm telling you. Those were the good old days.

And let me remind you of some other good old days. How about the Makawao dump, folks? Man, I used to love the Makawao dump – or the Makani "landfill" as it was officially called, although I'd rather call it a dump.

'Cause that's what we used to do. Dump. You and me. We'd throw anything in the back of the truck. Everything. Dirt. Plywood. Drywall. Used oil filters. Dead dryers. Dead cats. Dead TVs. Dead anything. Just drive up, dump, drive away. Cool.

But if you call it a "landfill," you can't have as much fun. Use that name and you have to remember that you have filled the land.

You can drive away. You can think about other things. But your dead poop remains.

And you and I pay to own that poop-filled land! It costs us six to seven MILLION dollars to get one 15-acre working dump, and one of those might last for three years at the rate we're dumping, and then a skin of dirt goes over it all. And then for 30 years – yes, I said 30 years – we, or our kids, pay to have the place monitored for leachate (stuffs that drip down) and methane (stinks that drift up).

So, 30 years from now, when I'm a rotten old geezer, people on Maui will be paying top dollar so that some expert can babysit my useless old poop.

I remember my last trip to the dear old dump, where the

wind blew grit in our teeth and the white egrets would rise up out of the stench whenever the earth quaked under the weight of the back-beeping earthmoving metal disasters that were tearing the land apart.

May 2, 1992. I know that date. It was the exact day after the Makani land... after the dump had closed forever and without my permission.

That day for some reason, in the innocence of my stupidity, I loaded my truck – a white, rotting old V-8 Chevy three-quarter-ton pickup – to the point where I was pretty sure I wouldn't get a ticket but, though I wouldn't admit it to you or anyone, I wasn't really sure.

Not totally.

In that load that day, you could sense some bad stuff. There were petroleum products on the move. There were organics slowly stirring back to life – only this time in a different form. There were steel beds and file cabinets, two apartment-sized washing machines. Instant fossils.

I was like the *Exxon Valdez* pushing itself up Kaupakalua Road on bald tires.

And then I reached the locked gate at the former dump. A pitiless sign informed me that this was now a "landfill" and that my Makani landfilling privileges had been revoked forever. Blown away with the "makani," the winds of change.

As my Portuguese neighbor had warned me that one day, about a year before, when I'd been up there sweeping the last bit of "fill" from back of the *Chevron Valdez* – the haoles had finally managed to fill up the dump.

So I headed off to the next closest dump, to the Kahului dump, saying wild and crazy things to myself in the cab of the truck, the load swaying with lots of sloshing and grinding, the gas gauge shaking down near the E. I got there all right, but I got there five minutes after they closed, and then I headed back Upcountry, not sure what fate lay ahead for *Moby Poop*.

The tire blew two miles up the Haleakala Highway.

Rush hour traffic screamed past like a fellow lunatic spitting tar hail into my face. I used the jack under that pile of you-know-what.

The spare tire was low on air, but I thought it might hold. I knew I was lucky to find a spare at all.

Soon it started to rain, and I believe it started to rain just as, one mile further up the highway, an engine rod kicked through the crankcase of that truck, and hot motor oil shot like heart's blood across what was suddenly an expensive piece of clever, though somewhat rusted, scrap metal.

As I stood there, half-paralyzed, leaning face-first against the side of my garbage pile, I couldn't imagine how I was going to get five tons of trash off of the side of the main highway of the most beautiful island on the planet Earth.

At one point I glanced all about me, and I saw sunshine and blue skies on every horizon, wherever I turned. The rain was dumping on me, only on me. Only on me and on my friend, the bride of Frankenstein. The rain was dumping.

Dumping.

The leachate dripped onto my dirty broken Adidas. The new methane stench rose into the air.

Listen. Nearly two million tons of total commodities are imported to Kahului Harbor every year. Close to 300,000 tons of trash get stuffed into the Kahului landfill every year. The Kahului landfill will overflow in two years.

My old truck held only a ton of that.

We live on a small island and we drink water that soaks through this small sponge of rock. We eat the food of this land, or at least we could.

This land has swallowed so much. Its lips have been pried open with shovels. And the land has made good of what we've given it, and the land pushes us upright, pushes us to attention.

When I take a handful of soil and breathe in its messages, I know I am home. I can smell my own best self. Our best selves.

I know the land will grow toward what we plant. After all, what we plant is an investment.

We need street-side pick-up of every manufactured product that we can possibly send back to North America. Send it back when we're done with it.

Make an agreement. When things break down, we send them back.

And hey, manufacturers, no need to pay us for the service. We'll accept the charges. We won't even complain when we have to go out and buy another washing machine or lawn mower or rake; we won't ask you why we should pay to replace your short-lived products.

If you live in Ha'iku, you never blame anybody for the fact that things rust, turn to compost, join the soil, become part of our lives.

We are what comes from our own soil. That's how we live.

Skinny-dipping can lead to other, more serious crimes

Parents, keep this article out of the hands of children.

It exposes a shameless crime, a crime our leaders have seen as threatening to the very fabric of Maui society – threatening, in fact, to fabrics of any kind.

I'm talking about skinny-dipping.

Here are the rude facts. It's Saturday, August 5th, and you're looking at the front page of *The Maui News*. A man and a woman have been arrested for swimming without their suits in a natural pool somewhere between Hana and Keʻanae.

You can picture the scene. The waterfall. Ginger plants. The police car. The stern officer with his gun, his fists planted on his fully-clothed hips, saying, "All right you two, come out with your hands up."

"On second thought," he adds hastily, "never mind. Hands down is okay."

When the criminals appear in Makawao District Court, the judge blasts them: "I will not tolerate such actions!" He fines them fifty bucks each.

This fifty bucks (twice) is actually more money than you think. At the time that this crime occurs, the minimum wage is $1.40, almost one-fifth of the minimum today. That makes the fine more like $200 or $250 (twice).

The year is 1969.

Let me say it right now, because you're probably thinking it: Shame.

Shame. Shame. How could those people be so rude?

Most of us spend our entire lives trying not to look at each other's buns. And of course, the law protects our constitutional right not to look at buns. (I think that's covered in the Bill of Rights, along with our right to leave half-eaten boxes of popcorn on the floor of the movie theater after the show.)

And now here come these bad people, willfully creating a situation whereby innocent folks who are driving past might accidentally glance to the left and, without wanting it – AUWE! – glimpse those buns.

Okay. Now let's get to the interesting part. I want to know why *The Maui News* printed this story on the front page. I mean, front page news is for catastrophes and disasters: "Haleakala Erupts!" or "President Declares War on Drugs!"

Not, certainly, "Buns Bagged in Nahiku!"

Front page placement suggests that all Maui people should alert themselves to this story. Other front page stories from 25 years ago include occasional reports on Maui boys who are dying in Vietnam.

On that same day, July 5th, you see two other lead stories somehow related to the nudism-threat piece above.

In one, 14 people at Makena Beach are arrested by the police vice squad on the morning of July 3rd and sentenced to 30 days in jail. They have been trespassing. If they don't want to serve the 30 days, they can accept a plane ride back home. They can be banished from the kingdom.

The article calls these people "hippies."

The other lead story, same day, tells of the court cases awaiting the Peahi residents of "Banana Patch." The drop-out cruisers of Banana Patch have created a free-form, Gilligan's-Island village, and now they must face the authorities to answer charges of alleged violations of sanitary regulations, building and housing codes, and land use codes.

It's clear to anyone who's scanning this newspaper that Maui has a problem with hippies. In fact, the paper obviously ranks this public concern right up there with "Safe Boating Week To Be Observed Here."

Two weeks later, a new law makes hitchhiking illegal in Maui County. (It still is.) This ban on hitching comes two days after "Moon Day" – so declared by Mayor Elmer Cravalho on the famous day of the "giant leap for all mankind."

The next June, an actual rock that was captured from the moon goes on public display down at War Memorial Gym. The rock, a trophy of conquest sent out to the border tribes to convince them that the central authority is really quite bad-ass, draws a big crowd. (Some of you were there, I'm sure.) On Maui, the moon-rock viewing crowds are the largest in Hawai'i, larger even than on O'ahu – 5,172 in one day.

On that same day, Goro Hokama announces that he is seeking his NINTH term on the County Council. He will win, and he will manage to keep his okole fixed to that important seat of leadership for another 24 years, right up to the last election. (I mention this only to suggest that Maui County's style of leadership has not shifted significantly since the dire, community-poisoning events of 1969.)

And – here it is again. I'm still looking through the old papers, and right around Moon Day I find another nudie story. Six people get arrested for trespassing and for indecent exposure out at remote Honolua Bay on West Maui.

On the same day, a respected Upcountry leader speaks of the forces of evil that have destroyed the nation's moral fiber. He addresses a Memorial Day ceremony at the Veteran's Cemetery on Baldwin Avenue. The valiant Maui men who are buried all around this orator (he tells us) urge him to proclaim to all who will hear: "You, the living, have failed us."

The speaker has eavesdropped on the mutterings of the mortal remains from the soil beneath his feet, but the newspaper article doesn't tell us what kind of weird telephone he employed.

It just tells us this. We the living have failed to stop the "false prophets." And who are these false prophets destroying everything good and decent? This respected Makawao leader describes them poetically: "These modern pied pipers with their flutes pipe our youth down the indescribably evil and lonely roads of marijuana, heroin and the madness of LSD."

For over a year, the paper has been emphasizing lots of little stories about indecent exposure busts, long-hair trespassers, and Banana Patch hand-wringing, so we know who these pied pipers really are.

The hippies. They want our moon-rock.

Now we have what we needed, an effective group label. ("Hippie" works as well for this as Nigger, Moke, Pencil-Neck Jap, and so on.) The newspaper has popularized its version of the problem, and our leaders are making hateful, group-label speeches. Now we're ready for violence.

Next thing you see is a story titled "'Hippies Our Biggest Problem' – Williams," quoting the President-elect of the West Maui Business Association as saying that the group's "single, most important task is 'to make Lahaina less attractive to the hippies.'"

No one bothers to define the term "hippie," but who cares? Everybody knows what they've done.

Mayor Cravalho makes a gloomy speech about some "organized, overt movement... for the total destruction of the system and establishment of which I am a part." He says that, "These people will try to exploit any cause, real or imagined, which can divide the community."

(Now, 25 years later, Cravalho continues to serve this community in a variety of leadership positions.)

The Maui police freely admit to unconstitutional practices against anyone with long hair. For example, instead of issuing citations, the police routinely arrest and harrass "long-hairs" for minor traffic violations. No one objects, except a few gooey-eyed lawyers fussing about civil liberties. Long-hair lawyers. Everybody knows what they want to do.

And then THE STORY breaks. Five hepatitis cases. June 27, 1970. Originating in the Banana Patch.

Maybe.

The authorities now have a reason to get in there and number all their bones.

You see a photo of the police chief, a Hawaiian man in a suit who talks with two bearded, white hoboes in ragged clothes. The two white men have their hands clasped over their midsections, as if they are being arrested for skinny-dipping; they're telling the police chief that, vibrationally speaking, broccoli is higher on the chain to God than, say, an animal with a bad attitude, like an anteater for instance. The police chief is imagining kicking their brown buns onto a Navy cargo transporter that will drop them off in Barrow, Alaska.

By early August, cases of hepatitis and dysentery start cropping up around the island. Despite citizen protests that government sources are giving false information, the mayor, the Department of Health, and the newspaper make it clear that the hippies, all of them, have diseased the people of Maui.

No one asks why our public health safeguards are so inadequate that a single case of hepatitis can spread throughout the community. No. No one stops to say, "Now wait – if some poor Portuguese man got hepatitis, would we brand all Portuguese as enemies of the people?" No. The problem is simple. It's the hippies, and everyone knows a hippie just by looking.

So, on August 29, the first violence is reported. Innocent people using Kalama Park are beaten and chased off with machetes and revolvers. Tourists camping in the Kihei area are frightened away.

The attackers are termed "locals." The attacked, "hippies." No one questions what those terms mean.

Again let me say it. Shame on those rude people who disregarded social customs and took off one-too-many articles of clothing while conjuring up their banana-patch villages and adam-and-eve frolics.

Notice, however, something else. Group hatred was sanctioned in 1970 by the leaders of this community. The aloha spirit grew sick. Of all the petty crimes of those years, this one offends me most.

And that's the naked truth.

THE PAST

Infectious diseases made us what we are today

As King Kamehameha XXVI recently pointed out, the united territories of "The Aloha Bloc" now exert more influence on this planet than any political power in the recorded history of the human race.

It doesn't matter how you measure – in square miles, number of citizens, military advantage, wealth, or knowledge. No nation has ever come close to the present success of the Commonwealth of Greater Hawai'i.

Islam and China, our two rivals for world power today, have both grown slowly over long histories of cold-blooded empire building. But Greater Hawai'i, which includes the entire Pacific Basin, Australia, most of Southeast Asia, more than 1/2 of both North and South America, as well as colonies and small member nations in both Europe and southern Africa, has taken only 200 years to grow to this size.

Two centuries ago, Hawai'i consisted of no more than 800,000 souls living in total isolation from the rest of the world. At that time, the English (Hawai'i's "discoverers") were set on a course to dominate the world. Rich with their clever Industrial-Revolution toys and tools, they were exploring and capturing new lands all around the globe.

Of course, the idea of a "British Empire" seems ridiculous today. Here in the last decade of the 20th century, England is a depressed colony of Saudi Arabia. The small remaining population of native Brits is a textbook case of an oppressed aboriginal race – impoverished, illiterate, and malnourished. The English language may well be dying out.

For another example of a global "wannabe" that never was, look at the backwards little United States. The 13 colonies had already declared their independence from England two years before Captain Cook arrived in Hawai'i. It didn't take more than 10 years to lay the foundations for a strong government designed along Greek and Roman models. They began to think about expanding westward.

Within 50 years, however, their government had all but collapsed. The will to expand, or even to resist invasion, seemed to abandon these newly-invented people.

Today the U.S. remains 13 small, bickering colonies hemmed in by the vast, thriving native American cultures, the thundering herds of bison, and the undamaged American wilderness which is protected and managed by the kahuna councils of the Hawaiian Commonwealth.

And how did these historical changes come about? What caused the collapse of the Western world and the meteoric rise of tiny Hawai'i to global prominence?

We like to think that these dramatic changes were caused by the natural superiority of the Hawaiian world view. After all, the kapu system is just plain practical, logical, and humane. Of course we like it best.

And yet, other systems do have their merits. I know it's hard to imagine, but democracy, capitalism, communism, or some other philosophy could have come to dominate the world.

We tend to assume that Hawaiian spiritual practices offer the only truth, that other religions are confused and foolish. We're accustomed to the sight of our stone temples, our heiau, throughout the world. We're comfortable with the fact that our annual Makahiki festival is now a global tradition, even in Muslim and Buddhist lands.

In our bellies, though, we know better. We've been taught not to be so narrow-minded. We know that all religions are founded in truth. Any one of them (even Christianity!) could have come to dominate our lives.

People do not give up their beliefs lightly. Remember how many Hawaiian missionaries were slaughtered by the frightened natives when they brought the good word to Christian nations in the Americas and Europe.

No. The Hawaiians dominate now – but not necessarily from any innate betterness. They dominate because of good luck. To put the matter bluntly, the early Hawaiians simply didn't die.

They had better immune systems than the English.

Hawai'i now rules the world because of a disease, a virus. The Last Laugh, they called it – though it was anything but funny.

Remember. When Captain Cook arrived in Hawai'i, his sailors brought diseases. Wherever Western people traveled, their diseases destroyed whole societies. Syphilis, smallpox, cholera, chicken pox, measles, and other fatal illnesses were wasting rival cultures.

In Peru, for example, 9 million people had welcomed the strange-looking white men. In less than 50 years, 93 percent of these people were dead. The few survivors could hardly resist the spread of Western culture.

The same collapse occurred even in Tahiti, where 75 percent of the people sickened and died over a 25 year period.

People of the West believed that their success was created by God; in fact, it had been caused by germs.

The tables turned when Cook arrived in Hawai'i. Though he brought all the white diseases, none of them proved to be a wide-scale problem for people living in these islands. Kahuna still do not agree about the reason for this immunity.

Ironically, though, Cook's men contracted a disease in Hawai'i, a totally new disease to which they had absolutely no resistance. The Last Laugh.

Soon after his one visit to these islands, while heading onward to explore the Pacific Northwest, Cook observed several of his crewmembers falling prey to this strange new disease. As Cook's badly-spelled logbook says, "Theyr sides shaike, their faces contorting unto ungodly smiles, and they gaspe as if laughing, where unto they meet theyr oblivion and are dead."

The disease spread quickly among the crew, and nothing in the ship's infirmary could be found to prevent it, or even slow its shark-like attacks. Many of the healthy crew members abandoned their tasks and lay on the ship's deck, paralyzed with terror and waiting to die. Stunned, Cook chose to turn back for England. All along the route of that desperate flight, Cook's men chuckled their way into heaven. The dwindling crew abandoned one of their two ships in Tierra del Fuego, then made a mad dash to the Thames.

Cook himself howled to eternal rest near the coast of Spain.

In the end, only 23 crew members returned to the streets of London, and the rapid decline of Western culture can be measured in quick, hilarious blooms of death that spread outward from this moment in London to Europe and to all its creations.

Let's be brutally honest. Suppose one tenth of the people you know suddenly die. It's a shock. Everyone's rattled, anxiety-ridden. You would find yourself at the heiau more often, making sacrifices for one reason or another. But suppose things get worse. Suppose, ten years later, nine out of every ten people you know have vanished in agony (including all your kahuna). You wouldn't believe it. In fact, you wouldn't believe anything. Disbelief would flood every crevice of your life. Faith would dart like a desperate rabbit for any hole or shade or shelter.

With every death, you lose some portion of your spirit. When 93 percent die, then only 7 percent of your faith remains.

If Hawai'i had lost even half that number of its people, then we might be living today in islands dominated by Western traditions and government. The native people here might be just as demoralized and frightened as the pathetic Brits are today in England.

Life could have been far different.

Let's not forget that any spot on the human earth has the potential to become the attention of the world, a source of great ideas, the belly-button of our species.

I know this sounds far-fetched, but depressed little towns like London, or even Washington DC, all have this potential. With luck, they too could attain the glory of a place like Makawao, which is today, truly, the "center of the universe."

Kamehameha's trade, white trash, and the Taro Festival

It's spring of 1994, and American troops are pulling out of Somalia, taking with them their motorized and electronic gadgets and their supply streams of Corn Flakes, Pop Tarts, paper towels, nudie magazines, disposable razors, Spam, microwave popcorn, raspberry jam, pocket calculators, pump-action toothpaste dispensers, Ray-Bans, and Snoop Doggy Dogg CDs. As a matter of fact, all WHITE soldiers are leaving. (Europeans, Canadians, like that.) The remaining U.N. troops come from Third World countries, and their trash is worth almost nothing.

For the past couple of years, thousands of Somalians found prosperity by "redistributing" the contents of the white soldiers' dumpsters. The rubbish of our officers, in particular, has turned quite a few locals into Mogadishan millionaires. Now, as politics shift and troops come and go, the black market trash industry is collapsing.

Only white people toss out valuable rubbish.

(Please forgive me for equating First World countries with "white people." Our troops contain people of all sorts, of course, so here's yet another example of a stupid group label. Nevertheless. Somalian trash merchants rate their garbage sources "white" when they mean, like I do, the culture of pink men.)

I heard about the trash merchants of Mogadishu by listening to public radio. That was on Monday morning. I'd just come back from Hana and the second annual Taro Festival. The coincidence got me thinking about our own history and the fact that, even though we ourselves come and go, our trash remains and leaves its mark on the generations that follow.

It's safe to imagine that no African man will ever feel quite the same about local politics after eating a blueberry Pop-Tart while staring at a nearly-naked picture of Cindy Crawford. The same change happened here, too, in 1778, when white people's trash dropped like a bomb into Hawaiian culture.

Not that Captain Cook HAD a lot of trash. He certainly wasn't setting up dumpsters on every new shore; his men weren't hurling out bulging Steel Sacks full of empty beer bottles and broken toasters. No. But the Hawaiians did find a great, culture-rocking wonderment in Cook's few remainders.

Nails, for example.

Nails were the first haole trash items, for which the locals traded pigs and sweet potatoes. Cook sighted the island of Kaua'i first, and he brought his two ships close to the coast near Waimea. There, in a scuffle over nails, a Hawaiian was given, instead, a different little piece of metal – a ball shot from a gun. Of the countless Hawaiian deaths brought about by white trash, this was the first.

I've taken this information from *The Life of Captain James Cook*, a big, fat door-stop of a book written in the early 1970s by J.C. Beaglehole. Beaglehole tells all, and I've picked through the stories to find out exactly what trash the good discoverer and his crew left behind.

The seas were rough off Kaua'i. Looking for shaky anchorage, the *Resolution* and the *Discovery* crept around to the west shore of Ni'ihau. They needed fresh water. A landing party led by Cook's first lieutenant, a chap named John Gore, was sent to Ni'ihau. Then a storm blew in, and the white men were forced to stay on shore for two nights.

This group dropped off another significant piece of Western trash – venereal disease.

To Cook's credit, he was upset about this particularly devastating deposit. It was, he wrote, "the very thing... that I had above all others wished to prevent." He had refused to let his men stay overnight on shore, but the storm thwarted his will. He meant well.

Clerke, captain of the *Discovery*, blamed it all on their "white trash" crew. "Our Seamen are in these matters so infernal and dissolute a Crew that for the gratification of the present passion that affects them they would entail universal destruction upon the whole of the Human Species."

A nail, a bullet, and the love-killing disease. Cook and his folks took little in exchange – water and food staples. They gave the Ni'ihauans some goats, pigs, and seeds "of the English breed," none of which survived the next year. Discouraged by continued stormy weather, the white folks then set off for the Bering Sea.

Nine months later, Cook returned from Alaska, and he spotted Haleakala first. He "lay to" along our North Shore. (The first European to see Ho'okipa!) Then he let the current carry him against the trade winds along the coast toward Hana. He had in mind rounding the eastern end of Maui to seek shelter on the leeward coast. One sight of the Big Island, though, convinced him to cross the channel.

If not for that decision, he might have landed in Kaupo or Kahikinui, where huge populations of Maui people fished, grew sweet potatoes, and managed the vital shipping traffic passing back and forth along that now ghostly and ecologically devastated stretch of this island. Instead, he brought his trash to Kealakekua Bay.

And there begins modern Hawaiian history.

On Hawai'i, the Englishmen gave whatever they felt they could in exchange for the heaps of supplies that the Hawaiians were letting them take – which included the entire fence surrounding the heiau (the temple) along with most of the carved images. The English needed firewood.

In exchange, Cook had the blacksmith fashion a little metal toolbox as a gift for the great chief Kalani'opu'u.

When an old seaman named Will Watman died of a stroke, they buried his body at the foot of the heiau and nailed up a little sign. They used wooden pegs for nails. Metal ones wouldn't have lasted any longer than a roadside mirror on a Ha'iku curve.

(The one put up by the County next to my house: 45 minutes.)

These were fine gifts, I suppose, but the Hawaiians wanted more. They must have lost patience with the general stinginess of these first tourists. The locals started popping out nails wherever they could get them, even out of the ships themselves. The English considered this activity to be theft.

(Cook and his men, we suppose, were just "borrowing.")

Bad feelings escalated until Cook himself fired a rifle into the chest of a chief and then, in turn, was given a fatal stabbing to the neck – with an iron dagger, a piece of his own trash. Cook's bones and hands were buried at sea, Kalani'opu'u was given a red felt cloak in exchange for his feathered one, and Clerke ordered the surviving crews to sail away for good.

Three days before this sad event, the *Discovery's* captain had struck a bargain with a quiet but powerful young chief. The chief swapped his elegant feather cloak for a real prize – nine long iron daggers.

The young chief was Kamehameha. The trade was portentous.

Years later, Kamehameha got hold of an even more significant piece of trash – a cannon, along with two English seamen to shoot the thing. With that cannon he was able to blast the warriors of Maui back into ʻIao Valley in desperate and bloody defeat. Then he moved on to Oʻahu, and sovereignty.

Western trash had a holy allure for Kamehameha, but don't kid yourself that we are any less naive. In fact, Kamehameha's trade defines the rest of our history. It begins with nine long daggers and escalates to include the tons of metal rubbish and unexploded ordnance that litter the island of Kahoʻolawe, the I-beams in our tall buildings, the nuclear subs that visit.

The Hana Taro Festival looked to me like the celebration that Captain Cook interrupted when he sailed into Kealakekua Bay. I met young taro farmers, forward-thinking, beautiful people. If I'd offered them nine long daggers, or partnerships in a hardware store, or high-level positions in a new resort, they would have said no.

For some reason, we are now ready to make a choice that's different from Kamehameha's trade. I feel bad for the folks in Somalia. They may be facing 200 years of cloudy confusion as they sort through the garbage. But in Hana, Sunday, the sun shone. It was a beautiful day.

my feet keep imagining the rocks beneath the mud of Ke'anae

My older brother is deformed.

I was told to take care of him and keep the family together, and he would make sure that I would never go hungry. It bothers me to admit, though, that I haven't given him much attention lately.

His name is Kalo; he hangs out with the folks in Ke'anae and Wailuanui. When I drive to Hana, I stop at the overlook and see him down there. He looks happy enough.

I'm talking about the taro plant, of course.

You may not buy the "brother" story as unscientific, but I think science has its limits and I'll stick with the version passed along by the Hawaiians.

Unless the two brothers stick together, they say, the light of Hawai'i will fade to black. No resort development will ever get it lit again. They can pour concrete over the taro landscape; they can build a Grand Blatant Ke'anae Resort, with a gigantic bronze taro plant sculpture on either side of the porte cochere.

The county can pass laws preserving Hawai'i, but there will be nothing spiritual left to preserve unless you and I take care of the family.

So they say.

Now, when I stand on the Hana road gazing down at those fanned-out lava peninsulas that butt into the thundering surf, and I find myself staring at all the lo'i, the square-edged artificial marshes continuously flooded with cool mountain water and fattening with the flag-like rich green leaves of the taro, I think about these things.

How ironic that we get to stop our cars there and stare down at the old fields and the few people who still keep the old covenant. Why do we stare?

It's not just how pretty it all looks. We stare as if we're straining to understand an urgently yelled message in a foreign tongue. We are deaf; we see the lips move, but we can't quite hear.

And you people down there, the ones we're looking at, poor folks, you can't even take a leak in the backyard without the risk of being captured forever in the home video of honeymooners from Indiana.

I'm sure you'd rather be left alone. But you won't be. In 1927, prison laborers cut the "belt road" through, connecting Ke'anae with the real world. If you get the whim, you can drive to Burger King in just over an hour.

Every day, people stop and stare. They can see what you've got. You're not safe.

Nosy people like me write about you, pass along the hearsay. For example, when you work in the muddy taro ponds of Ke'anae, your feet work down to the bottom, and you can feel the bony tips of the 'a'a, the rough lava, underneath. So they say.

I haven't been able to get that idea out of my feet. I keep feeling it.

Have I lost a brother?

I never see him anywhere but with you. He used to be every-

where on Maui; everybody was his friend. I hear he gets over
to the West side now and then, out by Honokohau, and he's got
friends in Waiheʻe. That's about it.

Never comes Upcountry anymore.

Mom and Dad made a baby, called him Haloa. But he was
funny looking; he turned into a taro plant. They had a second
kid, called him Haloa, too. He was funny looking in a different
way, turned into a human being.

Mom said, "You two ugly boys better stick together, malama,
take care of each other. 'Cause if you don't, I don't know who's
gonna!"

So the two brothers traveled around the Pacific Ocean, taking care of each other. Life was good. So they say.

Kalo, the older one, used example to teach his ignorant little
brother how to live. He grew all his offspring, his ʻoha, the
smaller copies of himself, all around the main stalk. As many as
five generations of copies of himself. All these ʻoha together,
that's the ʻohana, the family.

When the family breaks up, that's good. The kids get out
from under the parent's shadow. Nothing is lost; everything is
magnified. This is the family story.

The saying goes: I maikaʻi no ke kalo i ka ʻoha. Judge the
goodness of the taro by looking at the sprouts. You learn a lot
about the family by looking at the kids.

In Hawaiʻi, the two brothers got along better than anywhere
else on the planet. One square mile of Hawaiian-style loʻi can
feed as many as 15,000 people. The Hawaiians grew 300 kinds
of taro, grew it anywhere there was water – in the windward
valleys, on rock and beach flats near stream systems, on leeward slopes that had even a little moisture, even in mulch pits
that they created on lava fields.

About 500 years ago, plenty of taro was grown in the hills
above Keʻanae peninsula, but the peninsula itself was barren.
The farmers used to come down to the flat lava spill to fish and
gather opihi and limu.

Their chief didn't want to leave well enough alone. He was caught up in a rivalry with the chief of the next district, Wailua. He wanted more impressive lo'i; he wanted to challenge the taro supremacy of Wailuanui. So he talked his people into carrying dirt down from the hills, flattening and covering the 'a'a flow on the peninsula. Gradually they built up the soil, formed the walls and irrigation ways that you now see from the lookout on the Hana road. They turned a sheet of solid rock into a beautiful watery garden district.

Wars raged in this area, bloody fighting between Big Island fighters and Maui defenders. During the 14th century, a huge war fleet landed here, and the warriors doubled back on foot to ambush the Maui troops in Hana. No one ever messed with the people of Ke'anae and Wailuanui.

No one was ever stupid enough to do damage to older brother.

In 1778, Captain Cook anchored the *Resolution* right off the shores of Wailua. Kamehameha, not yet the conquerer of all Hawai'i, went out from Wailua shore and spent the night on Cook's ship. This is still our history. It happened here.

Ever since the Hawaiians created those lo'i, hundreds and hundreds of generations of 'oha have been snapped off and replanted. Born again. The plants that waggle their green flags across the Ke'anae peninsula today must be, in fact, the very same plants that those clever farmers and water engineers brought down to the peninsula centuries ago. These are the same fields; this is the same earth that they carried. Gesture of planting the same. Harvest habit the same. The same life.

Kalo is to the Hawaiians what the buffalo is to the Lakota Sioux, what corn is to the Hopi, the acorn to the Pomo, reindeer to the Laplanders, and (I suppose) the drive-thru burger to the Americans.

The everything symbol. The sine qua non. The without-which-there-is-nothing.

Is there any purpose to taro anymore, now that we have

instant mashed potatoes? Have cattle replaced the need for the buffalo? Does a White Leghorn do for the Bald Eagle?

You learn a lot about the family by looking at the kids.

A string of newspaper stories I'd dearly love to read

First one. Monday's paper.

Weirdness in Hana. Cop Vanishes.
Has Kaʻahumanu Returned?

Sightings of the ghost of Hawaiʻi's former ruling chiefess Kaʻahumanu had tongues wagging in Hana on Sunday morning. Rumors spoke of mysterious flashing lights on Hana Bay and the strange disappearance of two people, one of them a police officer.

No official explanation has been offered for the unusual events, reported by several witnesses.

Police and civilian search parties have scoured the greater Hana area since dawn hoping to locate the missing policeman and a Paukukalo teenager.

"We search this way out past 'Ohe'o and that way almost to Ke'anae," said Hana fisherman Abe Nakabuchi. "Never find nothing."

The missing officer was last seen at the eastern end of Hana Bay around 12:30 a.m. Saturday. Unexplained lights, apparently coming from the back side of Ka'uiki Head, had drawn a small, late-night crowd of the curious. The on-duty policeman was responding to calls of alarm about the lights.

These lights were bright, man," said one witness, a ceramist from Idaho visiting the Hana area. "Like fireworks, only you couldn't see where they were coming from. I still don't know what was going down."

The policeman was last seen walking on a cinder footpath that rounds the eastern end of the bay.

Another witness, a lobster fisherman from Nahiku, said, "He ask us what's happening here. So I tell him. Those lights coming from Ka'ahumanu cave. Had to be. So he go.

"I could see his flashlight shining. He stay going around the pu'u. Then right where that cave is, boom. Drums start up. Hawaiian style. Loud.

"Get chicken skin just talking about it."

At about the same time, 17 year old Deeanne Pejoria jumped from the truck where she had been parked along with three other teenagers. Witnesses say that she ran up the trail impulsively, ignoring the cries of her friends.

One of the friends, Rudybellinda Kipikipihiwi, said, "Then everything got real quiet. Even I stopped screaming. We could hear a voice, but we never catch the words."

Deeanne never returned.

Authorities may be baffled, but local residents express no doubts that these events mark the return of Hana's most famous former citizen.

Ka'ahumanu, the favored wife of Kamehameha I, governed the kingdom of Hawai'i from 1819 to 1832. She dismantled the kapu system, the rules and regulations through which the ruling chiefs expressed their power. When the missionaries arrived one year later, Ka'ahumanu set the stage for modern Hawai'i by publicly embracing Christianity.

She was born a refugee of war in a cave on Ka'uiki Head, the cinder hill which forms the right flank of Hana Bay. A brass plaque marks the spot.

"Some of us has spoke to her," said one informant who did not want to be named. "She says she changing her mind now. She made a mistake.

"Back then, she'd like us learn all the haole ways. So, how much did we learn? Choke I tell you. Enough already."

Second one. Tuesday's paper.

"Ka'ahumanu" Hijacks Ka'ahumanu Center. Liberty House Becomes Battleground.

A woman posing as Ka'ahumanu succeeded in driving the customers and employees out of Ka'ahumanu Shopping Center and into the parking lots yesterday afternoon. She and her followers then seized control of the Liberty House department store.

Police have cordoned off the entire shopping center and are attempting to negotiate the surrender of the woman claiming to be Hawai'i's former kuhina nui.

"I don't think she's planning to come out," said police spokesman Detective Hercules Silva. "She claims this is her Center. She's placed a kapu on all the stores."

"Ka'ahumanu" arrived at Ka'ahumanu Center without warning at about 10 a.m., accompanied by an estimated 30 to 40 followers, at least a dozen of whom are muscular "warriors" bearing authentic-looking ancient Hawaiian spears and clubs.

Frightening the customers with harmless but vivid flashes of light and the threatening gestures of her followers, she managed to clear the Center within 15 minutes. No one was hurt, and no buildings were damaged.

Thinking at first that the disturbance was a pro-sovereignty demonstration, police called on leaders of the Hawaiian community for assistance.

"Everyone said they didn't know nothing about it," said Silva. "But they all wanted to go talk with her. At first we let some of them in [to Liberty House], but they never come back out. Now we get plenty people, all kinds, wanting to go in there and join her, but we not letting anybody in."

All communication with "Ka'ahumanu" has taken place through her translator, a teenage girl from Paukukalo named Deeanne Pejoria. Pejoria was reported as missing when she vanished from Hana Bay on Saturday night. Dressed now in traditional kapa cloth, she no longer responds to her name and speaks only for the woman claiming to be the chiefess of old Hawai'i who died in 1832.

At one point during the police seige, Pejoria stepped out from Liberty House to deliver a message from Ka'ahumanu to the people of Hawai'i:

"I am in the House of Liberty. Why am I not free? And where are my free people? Why do they not come to me? I ended one kapu system. The time has come to end another one.

Before, we needed to learn from the haole. Our people were dying. I thought it was our only hope, to get as much of their mana as possible. But where are my people today? Who has survived? Who among you is maka'ainana, a true child of the land? Ka'ahumanu asks this question."

Witnesses reported hearing only one comment in English from "Ka'ahumanu" herself, an observation that broke from her lips when she first saw the bronze statue dedicated to the shopping center's namesake.

She asked, "Who that fat old tutu?"

Third one. Same day, page five.

Identity of Missing Policeman Revealed.

The Maui Police Department today released the identity of the officer missing since Saturday night. Detective Hector Ito of Pukalani vanished at Hana Bay while investigating mysterious lights flashing near the birth-cave of Queen Ka'ahumanu.

One police search party continues to comb the greater Hana area....

Fourth one. Wednesday's paper.

Ka'ahumanu Imposter Lashes Out at Costco Site.
Mob of Followers Grows Steadily.

Accompanied by an ever-increasing swarm of followers, the Hawaiian woman who claims to be the returned spirit of Queen Ka'ahumanu left her hideaway in the Liberty House store at Ka'ahumanu Center. She led a noisy and destructive attack on the construction site for Maui's newest high-volume discount store, Costco.

Her principal weapon is a 14 foot cannon, with which she blew enormous holes in the 300-foot long cement block wall intended to hold up the south wall of the new store. One antique specialist who saw the cannon close-up claims it to be at least 200 years old, of a type very commonly found on British frigates and warships.

Instead of cannon balls, the ragtag army fired pieces of the bronze statue of Ka'ahumanu that had recently been installed in the central courtyard of Ka'ahumanu Center. Witnesses say that the queen's head was the first body part to be used as artillery. When it pierced the enormous Costco wall, a cry rose from the mob of followers, who then used bulldozers and hand tools to create chaos at the job site.

Police stood by helplessly, having been ordered by both the mayor and by Governor Cayetano not to respond except to defend innocent lives.

"Until we know more about what we're dealing with here," said a spokesperson for Cayetano, "we'll be proceeding with a lot of serious reservations."

The self-proclaimed queen ended her 30 minute attack by walking with her estimated 200 or more followers up 'Iao Valley into the West Maui mountains. They have called for all the "real people" of Hawai'i to join them in a movement to "overthrow the haole kapu system."

Fifth one. Thursday's paper.

Missing Policeman Found at Remote Kaupo Site.

Detective Hector Ito of Pukalani, missing since his strange disappearance at Hana Bay on Saturday night, was found late Wednesday on a rocky beach in Kaupo. Mystified and confused, he could recall nothing about the 4 days of his absence.

"I don't know," he said. "I was walking around the corner at Ka'uiki Head. Then there was light. I don't know."

Detective Ito was found wearing nothing but the traditional-style Hawaiian loincloth, or malo. His uniform, gun, and other personal possessions are still missing.

Part II — the lies continue

First one. Friday's paper.

"Queen" Gathers a Royal Following
Hundreds Mass at 'Iao

They arrive with oversized coolers, chain saws, air mattresses, folding chairs, rice cookers, battery-run televisions. When they get to 'Iao, they're told to leave the modern contraptions behind.

"Bring food, hand tools, and one change of clothes," they are told. .According to rumor, weapons are being accepted, too.

An estimated 1,200 people have moved into makeshift campsites near 'Iao State Park, rallying around their queen – a woman who died 163 years ago and who returned to life, they believe, last Saturday night in Hana.

An unidentified woman who calls herself Ka'ahumanu has been the focus of numerous public demonstrations this week, including a two-day interruption of normal business at Ka'ahumanu Shopping Center and an outburst of vandalism at the

Costco construction site.

Authorities are still unsure what to make of this unexpected development. "We don't exactly know what she wants," said MPD spokesperson Detective Hercules Silva. "We don't know if this is some kind of hula festival or what."

Deeanne Pejoria, the Maui teenager who continues to speak for "Ka'ahumanu," has repeatedly delivered the following message:

"Queen Ka'ahumanu apologizes to the people of Hawai'i for her mistake in accepting the customs and values of the haole. She asks all her loyal subjects to re-dedicate themselves to Hawai'i nei."

People of all ethnic backgrounds have left their homes to gather in the West Maui mountains....

Second one. Same paper.

Stand-In Queen Can Expect A Bill.

Royalty has its price, and Ka'ahumanu will be asked to pay hers.

It won't be cheap.

As police and county officials hesitate, unsure exactly how to respond to the supposed return of the kuhina nui of old Hawai'i, the management of Ka'ahumanu Shopping Center is preparing for action.

The directors of Maui's biggest mall met today with representatives from Maui Land & Pineapple Company, Alexander & Baldwin, and the Costco corporation. The business leaders assessed damages and agreed on a plan that would help them recover the revenues lost during recent disturbances.

"We are prepared to·file a lawsuit against Ka'ahumanu, if it comes to that," said Assistant Comptroller for Ka'ahumanu Center Helga Nokidoki. "We're hoping that the queen will respond reasonably, however, to a fair demand for compensation."

Third one. Sunday paper.

Monster Demands Will Pay Off State Deficit
Queen Gets Bill For $350 Mill

. .Kaʻahumanu was happy to make amends. But that was before she glanced at the bottom line.

In a dramatic confrontation, the so-called queen of Hawaiʻi and hundreds of her followers met yesterday with representatives from Kaʻahumanu Center, Maui Land & Pine, A&B Commercial Properties, and Costco.

The queen offered a formal apology to the business leaders and promised to "hoʻopono," to make amends for damages to the Costco wall. She was struck speechless, however, by the unexpected size of the sum being demanded.

The queen walked proudly in the front of her followers, many of whom have adopted traditional Hawaiian garb. At six feet tall and heavily tattooed on her legs, hand and tongue, eyes flashing and wild hair moving in the gusty winds of ʻIao Valley, Kaʻahumanu made an imposing, regal figure. She and her close advisors were dressed in kapa cloth stamped with intricate designs and draped with garlands of maile, ti and other greenery.

The royal procession met head-to-head with its opposite, a long line of bureaucrats dressed in conservative business attire, most of them carrying laptop computers, briefcases, ledgers and file folders stuffed with accounting sheets. The leader of this entourage was Assistant Comptroller for Kaʻahumanu Center Helga Nokidoki, a thin, gray-haired bookkeeper from Indiana who moved to Maui only five years ago.

Nokidoki listened to Kaʻahumanu's offer to make amends, smiled slightly, then announced the payment due as $350 million.

Explaining the large sum, Nokidoki named the damage to the concrete wall, destruction of a "timeless monument of public art," loss of income for the entire shopping center over a two-day period and irreparable damage to the mall's public image.

No one wants to shop at Ka'ahumanu Center if they think someone like Ka'ahumanu could show up at any time," said Nokidoki.

When asked how these figures were derived, Nokidoki said, "We follow certain formulas. It's too difficult to explain."

In an unexpected twist, Nokidoki and her team announced that they would donate the queen's payment directly to the state treasury in order to compensate for the recently-announced shortfall of $350 million.

Could it be anything more than sheer coincidence that Ka'ahumanu's debt exactly equals the state's shortfall? When asked her opinion, Nokidoki repeated her earlier comment, "We follow certain formulas. It's too difficult to explain."

Divided equally among Ka'ahumanu's estimated 2,000 followers, the bill comes to $175,000 per person.

Fourth one. Monday paper.

Queen's Followers Vow To Work Off Debt.

"The life of the land is preserved in righteousness."

These words translate our state motto, once coined by a Hawaiian king:

"Ua mau ke ea o ka 'aina i ka pono." Quoting this phrase, Ka'ahumanu and her roughly 2,000 followers . . . . announced today that they would work "no matter what it takes" to pay off the collective debt of $350 million.

The county responded immediately by arranging positions in a wide range of programs for public benefit, including security guard work, roadside clean-up crews, yard maintenance teams for resorts and condominiums, janitors in public facilities and parking supervisors at the Kahului Airport.

Queen Ka'ahumanu herself will serve as the custodian at Kamehameha III School in Lahaina.

Conservative estimates show that the debt will be fully paid in as soon as 11.6 years.

"Above all," said a spokesperson for Ka'ahumanu, "the people of Hawai'i must ho'opono. They must do what is right."

Fifth one. Almost exactly one year later.

Ka'ahumanu Spotted At Homeless Shelter

The woman popularly believed to be the resurrected spirit of Queen Ka'ahumanu was spotted standing in line for a hot meal at the Homeless Shelter yesterday.

"I know it was her," said Deeanne Pejoria, a Paukukalo teenager who volunteers once a week at the shelter. "I see that tongue with all the tattoos. So trippy!"

Several good reasons NOT to be here now

Take a deep breath. Now hold it.

What are the chances that you just breathed somebody else's air?

Let me be specific. You just sucked in a bucketful of air; officially, these molecules are now part of you. What are the chances that ONE molecule of this lungful was once a part of Julius Caesar's dying breath – the official last gasp of the founding henchman of the great Roman Empire as he was shishkebobbed simultaneously by dozens of his own political cronies? Do you think it's even possible?

Could you and Julius be so intimate as to share the same molecule? Imagine – for a while, the molecule hung out in his earlobe, and then he exhaled it, and now it's circulating around in your kidneys, and tomorrow it'll be in somebody's bananas – like that? What are the chances?

Ninety-nine in a hundred.

That's what they say. In fact, the odds are extremely good that you just sucked in a tad of old Julius right this moment.

Okay. You can let it out.

Two things happened to me today. I saw in the paper that Bumpy Kanahele, the Hawaiian sovereignty leader, has been arrested without bail for refusing to respect the civic authority that invaded his kingdom about 100 years ago. He could be sentenced to 5 years in prison. They're refusing bail because Bumpy used angry, threatening language and frightened the representatives of the civic authority.

Now for the second thing that happened, and it happened right after: I suddenly remembered this weird fact about breathing and Julius Caesar and the rest of it.

I even remembered where I'd read it, so (with some difficulty) I looked it up it again – in *What Counts*, a wonderful paperback collection of all the mind-jolting facts and statistics that *Harper's* magazine publishes each issue in its "Harper's Index" column. I remembered right.

With every breath, you breathe in a million pasts.

And directly above this strange fact, *What Counts* lists an even more curious statistic. It tells us how long "now" lasts.

Think about it. The present moment. It does exist, at least in our minds. If it exists, it must exist for a certain length of time. How long?

Here's another way to ask the question: if you think, "Oh, I'm really happy right now," how much time do you give yourself before you can start to feel insecure again? Or, when your boss (whoever he or she may be) says, "Do it now!" – how much time have you got before you begin to look deliberately unwilling?

"Harper's Index" says, "Estimated number of seconds that humans perceive 'the present' to last: 3."

One. Two. Three. Yep, that sounds about right to me.

The grand slogan of my generation was always, "Be Here Now." I still hear people say it. I think I heard Bill Clinton say it the first time somebody shouted out, "Hey, what about that Whitewater investment?"

America is a very "now" culture, and Hawai'i never has been. Therein lies the dynamic of our lives.

Three seconds. Be here now, and that's all you get.

Suppose you actually COULD achieve the state of total be-here-now-itude. If you DID live totally "for the moment" – and if you didn't weenie out – I think you'd want to drive your car as fast as you could off a sheer cliff on the road to Hana. You'd be willing to blow yourself up, and the whole world around you, just because you'd disrespect the past and future so vehemently.

I can't "be here now," and this is where I separate from my many wonderful spiritually-minded friends. Many of them keep clutching and shaking their "now" like a big, noisy Christmas present. They believe that they truly aren't... whatever it is that they THINK they aren't. Some even believe that they aren't really named whatever they THOUGHT they were named.

But I could never change my name. To me, anymore, the past is just too fundamental.

My breath, my face, my thoughts, my community have all been delivered to me out of the huge past, and I can only reshuffle the ingredients to whatever extent that I can work my puny will power. I am all that I am made of, and all that I am made of has been shared around the planet with everything.

We're all just walking puffs of Caesar's breath. We're all a bunch of mad gardeners trying to keep up with the pruning. I don't believe that we create the plants and the soil.

My garden has real trees, not crystal nectar fountains. When I walk across the lawn, that's real dog poop I try to dodge. I don't mind acknowledging the past. The past is awesome and full of mystery.

I once had the chance to walk into the heart of a Neolithic temple over 5,000 years old. Newgrange, it's called, in Ireland. A "passage grave." Essentially, it's a man-made hill twice the height of a 2-story house and as wide as a football field, created by Stone Age people who cleverly stacked up an incredible number of unliftable boulders. These unknown builders decorated their special hill with a skin of bright white quartz stones, and they carved beautiful spiral designs into the raw rocks.

But that's just the beginning. When they built the hill, these skillful "cave men" left a passageway into the center, so they could stoop and crawl their way along a 65-foot passage into a secret chamber at the very heart of their hill. The hollow chamber is 20 feet high and big enough for a dozen people to stand upright. These builders also left three very short passages that spur out from the central chamber – three chapels, so to speak, almost like windows in a museum display. In each of these chapels they placed a hand-ground, bowl-shaped rock containing human ashes and cremated bones.

Try to imagine the reasons those people felt such intense devotion. To whom? To some Julius Caesars of their own time.

But Newgrange is much more than a Flintstone mausoleum. It's also a cosmic clock. Over the entrance, where you have to squat and use your hands to squeeze yourself into the passage, the stone that scrapes your back is a very carefully chosen, long, brick-shaped piece. And above it the builders left a slit, a horizontal keyhole.

When the sun rises on the morning of the Winter Solstice, the very moment when days start to lengthen and winter begins to withdraw, that heroic first sunlight of the new year runs right through the keyhole, pours straight down the passage, and lights up the central chamber like a pine-pitch torch.

Science meets poetry meets history meets religion.

These people had very sophisticated methods for measuring, calibrating, and constructing. Not many of us slick, modern types could make something like Newgrange, no matter how many boulder-rolling brutes we had to help us.

Basically, I think we're afraid of the past. The human race, exactly as it is today, has been around a million years, and all that forgotten experience haunts us from our bones.

So we draw a veil over the past, and imagine that pre-history was populated by dirty dimwits who went around questing for fire. None of them could tell a joke or sing a song. We also draw a veil over living cultures that remind us of our monstrous past. In fact, we surround ourselves with these veils and hide. Just being here. Now.

That's a little like escaping from a mugger by slipping a number 56 shopping bag over your head.

The problem is this – just because something's past doesn't mean it's gone. We inherit the past just as surely as we inherit our elbows and our teeth and our noses. And if you don't take care of your teeth, you're an idiot.

Bumpy knows that.

During that same summer that I crawled into the Newgrange passage grave, I had an even more intimate experience of just how nonessential the "now" is.

I was with an old Irishman, and we were traipsing around on the slopes of Carrowmore, a wind-swept grassy hilltop near Sligo. We were in the heart of the land of the fairies. Across the valley, we could see the supernatural dome of a little mountain called Knocknorea. They say that once a year on a full-moon night a hidden door opens in the bottom of that hill, and out comes a procession of fabulous spiritual creatures led by the astonishing Maeve herself, the Faerie Queene. This parade of living memories then crosses the valley floor and disappears under a flat-topped mountain called Ben Bulben. The poet W.B. Yeats is buried near there, at his own request.

Well, this was late summer, the dry part of the year, but Irish rain – just as in Ha'iku – respects no season. Suddenly, the sky began to pelter us. We needed a shelter. The old guy said, "We can duck in here."

And what was it? Another passage grave, a somewhat shabby little thing, but big enough for us to huddle in there like two Cub Scouts in a pup tent.

I knew that cold rain was falling outside on the thick, thick walls of the little hill that sheltered me – though in the central chamber life was snug and dry. In the quiet of that Stone Age tomb, we could hear each other breathing, each of us sucking in more of Julius Caesar's air.

No doubt the fairies and ghosts were moving about in the rain, perhaps even the ghosts of those sophisticated Stone Age craftsmen who had assembled my haunted shelter.

My sense of my position in time began to slip, and slip cheerfully away. If it hadn't been for a few modern tokens – the ballpoint pen in my pocket, my belt-buckle – I might have come totally unglued, and walked out of that passage grave into any century, any past you can imagine.

Bumpy, if I were sitting in that little passage grave again today, the first person I would think of would be you.

THE PRESENT

Even the green grass is a stranger here, buddy

You are the person I admire, because you are a member of my tribe.

I stumbled after this thought – grabbed at it as a way to pull myself out of a terrible jam – last night while I was sitting outside. I don't know if you do this, but when I'm alone at night, I like to think. I try to remember HOW I think, after the phones shut up and the obligations pull back into the darkness to doze, until the early dawn gets them roused and howling and hungry again.

I dodge them by sleeping less.

But thinking can get you into trouble, and I admit it. Thinking can make you stutter, lose your wallet, change your name to something that no one wants to call you, stop eating what you like to eat, and forgive the unforgivable.

I was thinking about the grass around my house, and that's what got me started.

The grass around my house – and there's a lot of it, whatever tolerates the regular mowing and settles into something like what people from Los Angeles call a lawn – all of it came originally from seed that was brought to Maui in cattle feed on wooden boats that crossed the Pacific. And not very long ago.

I moved to Haʻiku for the sheer pleasure of blinding myself with the color and health of its green grass. I still remember my first sight of it, when I was driving a truck full of Lahainaluna students up Kokomo Road, though I can't quite remember when that was.

I feel that same rush of gladness every time I drive past Haku Baldwin's horse paradise, with its sky-blue stables, on the mauka side of Makawao Avenue, that same eagerness to give up half of my dreams just to be around that quiet groundfire of breathing green.

The first horses came to Hawaiʻi on the sailing ship *Lelia Byrd* in 1803, the same year that foreign diseases came and started slaughtering Hawaiians in every village and every household. The first cowboys from Portugal didn't arrive until about 100 years ago, and I really don't know when in that century my "lawn" arrived. Maybe one of you can help me with this.

I heard from a friend that the tall stand of pines crowning Giggle Hill – fat-trunked and pole-straight and nearly limbless, crowded in rows like corn – were planted by pirates as insurance in case they ever got dismasted. I still have a hard time imagining the work involved in dragging a new green mast covertly down the footpaths from Kokomo to the shore, maybe Pauwela Point, maybe Maliko Bay.

I've read that Kaʻuiki Head, next to Hana Bay, never had ironwoods, no trees, in the not-too-distant old days. I've heard that kiawe was introduced to force us to wear shoes. I understand that the deliberate introduction of the mosquito is a well-documented case. I'm over 40 now; I no longer think that any of this was a very long time ago.

All these thoughts felt important because the night air barely moved. Power was rising out of the soil.

Distressed with thinking about the acres of that upstart, malihini grass, I looked at other plants. The bananas were ready for anything, free now from the beating of the wind, too happy to actually care that they really belong in Malaysia or New Guinea. That they have no permission to be here.

All around me, the red ti plants were reaching for the most nearly unbearable union possible, their leaves bent in every possible attitude of yes. Their ancestors were brought here by Polynesians – or, perhaps, since they are red and ornamental, by some early 20th century housewife-horticulturist whose ancestors had come here from Massachusetts. I got them out of the dump. They are cuttings of cuttings of cuttings going way back. They are the very same plants that came here centuries ago.

And nothing was going to stop those red tis from enjoying this windless night.

I was sitting on the lanai, the floodlight falling on my lap. Three years before, I'd built the cottage myself with materials shipped to me from a home supply outlet on the northwest coast of North America – sticks and plywood from mills in the Rockies, stain from a factory in Bellevue Washington, nails from a foundry in Strongsville Ohio.

Most of my news comes from the cities of America. My shirt was buttoned up for the first time in Indonesia, and the Chinese had a hand in my trousers. The light that was falling on my lap burned down from hot, Mexican-made tubes fired by turbines that turn with burning black slick from Alaska. The truck I drive was shipped here on a barge.

We all like so much of what comes from distant places.

My golden retriever, Makapu'u, was almost completely manufactured, through breeding, by European people, now long dead, who placed a great premium on fetching something – I don't know what. Knowing my dog, I'd also guess that these people put another great premium on totally agreeable personalities. Makapu'u has almost no deeper wolf-nature, except when raw meat is involved.

He and I sat near each other on land that I "own" according

to the teachings of my tribe. Because I work hard and pay money, a bank and the local government agree that this is "mine." Having this land gives me freedom and loneliness, as my new gate indicates. The land I describe could hold a very small village, but such a village is forbidden by the rules of this tribe. I must be alone here, in my own boundaries.

Most of the rules of my tribe were brought here from the cities of the eastern shore of North America; before that, from Britain – the notion that I should "own" some land, for example, and the concept that I could "own" but not "ranch and eat" my dog. These rules define what I can't do with my natural desires.

Last night, sitting in the dark, I believed that it is the land itself, not us, who tries these things out. It's Haleakala, this mountain, that tries out a new coat of grass, a new group of people, a new set of tribal rules. The land is doing an awful lot of experimenting right now, and I try not to take these experiments too personally, nor too seriously.

But the tribe itself is personal. You, like me, are personal. We're all essentially homeless people enthralled with the home we use. We're all lucky to be here, and we know it, and I believe that each of us, deep down, somewhat begrudges the fact that nearly everyone else is here, too.

Last week I attended a session of the Maui County Planning Commission. The question came up: What is a Hana resident? One of the commissioners suggested the idea that Hana stopped being "Hana" when the mill closed down in 1944. The only true Hana residents are those people who were living in Hana more than 50 years ago.

Such an idea makes planning very difficult, given the dizzy pace of experimentation that this land has been enjoying during the past, brief 200 years.

None of us is sure – even though we dearly want to be – what the next move should be, or even if we have one. We're just starting to get ourselves organized here, and we don't even know what it is we've started.

In the silence last night, I could hear the soft roar of cars every so often getting close and going away. I always hope that they make the curve.

That driver is always someone I admire. Another member of our constantly possible tribe.

Don't worry about tsunamis, watch out for moonlight!

The big moon of October is bearing down on us like a full-armed barmaid from Bavaria, hoisting 5 brimming mugs in each hand high over the heads of the yelping and hollering crowd.

Where I live, the cows are yelling and bugling late into the night. I can't keep the lawn cut. Here, at the sagging rear end of summer, the plants are exhaling more than they're inhaling. The new leaves just can't belch fast enough.

My driveway is coated with smashed, fermenting guava fruits. Papayas, too. Yellow and orange fruit is rotting where it falls. The night air smells of jelly and dust. Large guava limbs have ripped away under the strain of their own weight and come crashing down. Banana stalks are toppling from the heaviness of their own sharp-ribbed fruit.

Along the roadsides, you see people fighting back against the heaving burden of leaves and branches. This is the month of mowers and Round-up and machetes, of road crews scraping the edges of the asphalt and glueing down new safety dots. Deep in the distant purple air, the general quiet is closed in by the faraway whining of chain saws.

Lots of mosquitoes. The stagnant ponds are thickening and swelling. We'll have mosquitoes till the first big gully-flushing rain builds up.

A fullness fills everything we do.

For the time being, we're just not worrying as much as. We have more than enough of. We've had our fill.

The whole atmosphere feels pumped up, as if we could see the long end of an enormous basketball-inflating needle sticking through the outside hull of the sky. Cats nearly everywhere have, or want to have, children.

This is the month of ripeness and forgetting.

The trade winds have died so often over the past couple of months that we're in danger of forgetting the future. Clapping mosquitoes to death is not exactly the way we want to be remembered, anyway.

Nothing can hurt us, anyway. Last week the whole island survived a terrible tsunami which turned out to be nothing but a society-stopping ripple, a hoax, an unplanned freak holiday in a month of freakish and dubious holidays – Halloween, Columbus Day.

According to the Hawaiian historian David Malo, we're in the last month of the season of Kau, the vegetable maximum before the sun begins its slow decline to the south. Scorpio is sprawling above the horizon, its flat head pointing directly at the setting moon. If we hadn't set fire to all our bridges that connect us with the Hawaiian past, Malo says, our Makahiki season would be starting now. Sometime soon (in the old way) we would be paying our taxes.

We would be caught up in a public display of giving away our treasures; we'd be handing over swine and feathers, new bark cloth and bundles of surplus poi wrapped between planks of smoke-dried shark meat.

This is the month when all of us have to unload our excess, so that we don't choke on it.

After all, Halloween is not really about spooks; it's about excess. The earth and its people have piled up a superabundance. Originally, it was not children who went door to door. The poor and the needy were the ones who would mask themselves, then pound on the doors of the abundant, yelling "Give it away! Come on! Unload!"

Halloween began as an old Irish festival of forced taxation: Disgorge, before you drown in all that! No one gets to sit and sicken on his hoard, not in the oozing overflow month of October.

For this is the dangerous month of satisfaction. To "satisfy" is to "make someone sad." I'm not making that up. I'm only reporting on the history of those words.

Watch out for satisfaction. The next step is coma.

In 1783, the first human being ever to leave the earth ascended 80 feet in the air for a 5-minute hot air balloon flight over Paris, France. Fourteen years later, another Frenchman stepped OUT of a hot air balloon that was more than 2,000 feet in the air. He was hanging onto a 23-foot diameter umbrella, thereby making the first parachute jump. Airplane inventor Wilbur Wright called this the most courageous act in aviation history.

The fact that this aerial pioneer succeeded only in pile-driving himself into a heap of *humain tartare* (or, as we say, sashimi) makes me question the precise use of the term "courageous." But I know why he jumped. I noticed the date.

Both of those stunts took place in the month of October, which makes total sense to me. October is the month to do the unreasonable and the impossible. Either that, or go crazy while you clutch your stash.

So have a garage sale. Donate. Walk up to strangers and give them things. Confess. Empty the refrigerator. Spay the cat. Get to the dump. Shave. Cut your nails. Walk up and down the roads singing at the top of your lungs.

You want to unload.

Otherwise, that fat-ass harvest moon's gonna come hauling itself up over Mauna Kea, then over the shoulders of Haleakala, then come pouring down, smothering down on you. And then you'll be too loaded-down to leap up out of its way. You might get trapped and smothered under an avalanche of moonlight, pinned there, conked out.

Then it'll take the thickest downpours of December to flush you free of that dream.

If you MUST have a personality, then please show it off

For What's-his-name

The date's already set for Saturday, June 3. We're going to have an annual festival for Ha'iku, call it the Ha'iku Flower Festival. I'm not sure how the idea got started.

But I think it's a good one.

I am curious to see all the people of Ha'iku in one place – stepping shyly forth from their gulches and banana patches and ranch houses and shacks, blinking and staring around at all the funny-looking strangers.

I'm telling you. A lot of saints and a lot of sinners. A group with lots of personality!

I could tell you some stories – but I won't. Not in the public press. Besides, this ain't no dot-dot-dot column.

Well, I might tell one or two.

Just to prove that Ha'iku has a lot of personality.

Because this festival has got to reflect the Ha'iku personality.

And what could THAT be? Well, it must be made up of all
Haʻiku people's personalities combined 50/50 with the larger
personality that we build without thinking by our collective
interactions – how we drive on the road and how we shop, what
kinds of businesses we own and to what degree our streets are
safe. That sort of thing.

The big question is this: what's gonna happen at the first
Haʻiku festival? What would suit the Haʻiku personality?

I imagine a titanic backhoe wrestling contest. Then an earthmoving competition. Have a race to tear up the Pukalani
bypass. Or dig tunnels under it.

Anything involving water – especially heavily moving water
or water that falls in large sheets – would allow us to show off
our acquired skills. A race pushing cars through chest-deep,
gushing floodwaters. A sand-bagging contest.

Create a 30-foot wide raging torrent and send it across somebody's property. Give each team six shovels, an ʻoʻo, four cases
of Budweiser, a telephone....

No. Too complex.

Run a cable across Maliko Gulch and let people zip across
with a pulley.

Of course, various demonstrations side by side would reveal
the many contradictions in Haʻiku's personality.

The animal butchering demonstration, for example, would
draw the crowds that the blue-green algae smoothie bar would
never miss. We'd need an air-brushed pickup truck and tinted-
windowed car show, of course, but I think we should also offer
an I've-dropped-acid car show, and set up a special booth for
the "Dare For Drive Slow" Society, with its bumper stickers and
buttons.

Please address your suggestions for Haʻiku Festival events to
Untested Ideas Editor, P.O. Box 1033, Haʻiku HI 96708. I need
your ideas because I just can't keep my attention on the problem. My mind is totally occupied by another train of thought –
I mean, what is "personality," anyway?

How did we get one? Where did it come from? Some people are born with more personality than others, apparently. Why is that?

Most of all, is a personality contagious? And if you've got one, can you take herbs for it or something?

I was raised with the idea that my personality came with me when I was born and it's going to stick with me even after my body drops. Think so? After I'm dead, no matter what happens – whether I'm stuck getting my punishment or I'm jumping from new body to new body – will my personality still be with me?

In the afterlife, will I still dislike cats?

Lots of people say so, Christians and Hindus alike. To them, we are who we are, dead or alive, whether we live in Haʻiku or drift like a gas from planet to planet.

But the other way to look at it makes more sense to me. In the other view, my personality is just one of my body parts, like my toenails or the way my hair smells. I lose it when I lose the whole package.

In this view, my soul does go on after I die, but my soul is no more different from your soul than any one frosted 60 watt light bulb is different from any other. Soul-wise, we're each just one more unit of the great cosmic goo.

The Elizabethans felt this way. They believed that the personality is a physical defect.

They believed that the personality is a problem you have with your body that you should correct by watching your diet and by taking herbs and things.

For them, the best people lack personality altogether.

The Elizabethans got this idea from the ancient Greeks, and they applied it to their practice of medicine. I'm speaking here about the people of England some 3 to 4 hundred years ago, Shakespeare's time, not very long ago at all – modern people who spoke exactly the way we do except with a kind of verve and a set of interests that we reserve for other purposes.

They also believed that gold is a shade of red.

That's how fragile our deeply-held beliefs can be.

Imagine what this means. Your personality, the "real you" that your best friend knows all about – your edginess, your fears, your excitements, what makes you laugh, what gets you horny, what gets you fighting mad, what makes you gloomy and withdrawn – these are symptoms of your uniquely diseased and imbalanced state.

According to the old belief, we each have four different kinds of fluid moving around in us, liquids sloshing and mixing between our gizzards and our intestines. Humors, they called them, as in the word "humid." Sloshing and oozing.

Each liquid drifts in a different direction. One makes us excited, one angry, one stubborn, and one depressed. These four juices mark the four extreme corners of the human personality.

Our personality is a circus running around between these four reactions: 1) manic and hysterically eager (sanguine), 2) explosively furious (choleric), 3) downright refusing to participate (phlegmatic), 4) exquisitely self-absorbed (melancholic).

The goal of the Elizabethans was to balance these fluids until the traits canceled each other out. If you've got all your fluids in perfect balance, none will stick out and make a fuss. You will live without any of the four extremes of personality. You will be good-humored.

I see good-humored people all the time – I think. Of course, I forget to notice, because these good-humored people have no personality.

I remember that one guy, though – what's-his-name.

Oh, never mind.

Thank God for good-humored people. Thank God for the guy who changes his name to "I. Breathed Yeast" and speaks very softly from that day forth. For shoppers who always have the right amount of change. For good people who are baffled by the stories they read in the newspaper. These people keep the world safe and competent.

I hope we'll have a special area for them at the Haʻiku Flower Festival. A booth for "Personality-Free People." These are spiritual people. They represent the soul, the soul that we will all, one day, be nothing else but. The 60-watt light bulb.

If I see a 60-watt bulb person running for political office, I always vote for her or him. I want only good-humored people in office writing bills that will restrict my freedom. I think I myself once hoped to become a 60-watt bulb.

I just can't seem to be friends with 60-watt bulbs. All of my friends have personalities.

They all have these defects, where one humor dominates another, and they have these wild swings – from raging fury to laughing at the top of their lungs, and then to thinking about what it all means and how ridiculous it all is, and from there to sadness.

Or they move in a different sequence. But they do move.

The pulse of their swings and their long resistances make up the painful and dangerous dance they dance – the cha cha cha of flesh and blood.

The good-humored man, by contrast, slips painlessly through, as if his life is teflon-coated.

The good-humored woman refuses to get involved in emotional outbursts. In that stillness, she makes room for a higher intelligence which guides her and those about her. She is a wet, jelly-thick lake of calmness and joy.

I don't think she lives in Haʻiku. I'm sure I've never met her. Or did I – nah. Can't remember. What's her name.

But let's set up a booth for the good-humored anyway, and see if we notice anybody showing up. The rest of us can snort and spit and belly-up to the bad-humored places with all the flashy fury and unexpected impulses that make me me, you you, and Haʻiku... well, Haʻiku.

Because these odd humors are not eternal. Therefore, they are precious.

The other morning I was out on the street, running. (I do that sometimes, to pay for my sins.) It was dawn. I came up to the top of a steep section of the street, a long grade that always makes my head spin and my blood panic. I was running straight into the just-risen sunlight. In front of me, on the roadside, I could see a butchered carcass.

The remains of a pig.

The bones were red where all the meat had been sliced away. The rib cage and keel stuck straight up into the morning sky, the thin, bacon-like tissue stretching like a veil across a striking black architecture of bones. Sunlight glowed through this thinly stretched flesh which shone with a serenely rich, rose-colored light. Almost a gold.

This was a terrible lampshade of life's precious beauty. Something to read by.

I'm all for celebrating personality, if only because it will be gone so soon.

Nothing this strong and good can truly pass from the world

I'm a mongrel just like most of you – the result of a lot of unplanned and random breeding. My ancestors, God bless 'em, seemed to like variety.

And who can blame them? They were common people, not blue-bloods, not purists. The whole human race was fair game to them, because they knew their place – right in the middle of it all, rubbing elbows with the whole furry human pack, no matter where they went.

I can understand why they didn't want to marry the girl or guy next door. What's the fun of smooching someone who looks, smells, and sounds just like you? Anybody can have that experience.

Just pull the covers over your head and start singing.

No. I think they liked the glamour of the thicker hair, the whiter skin, the browner eyes, the whatever-it-was that they themselves didn't have. They liked the eternal mystery of marriage to some foreigner, someone they would never ever really understand. They were probably life-long curious to find out what their cross-breed kids were going to look like.

Take my grandfather, for example.

He was a white man and he fell in love with a girl from an island race, from a people considered (until quite recently) savage, inferior, untameable.

He was of Yorkshire English stock, and he passed down that blunt name you see on the title to this book, the name that Hawai'i folks have such a hard time getting right – they always want to make it "Woods," I think because the real name seems to end too soon. I even have a jacket made in Hong Kong that has my name stitched inside: Paul Wooo.

He was a white man, I tell you, but he never sold rum to the natives, never broke a treaty, never swindled a brown man out of his land. He fought disease, he was a doctor. He had no office. He walked to his patients' houses, and he opened up the family parlor at night for the laboring people. When he died, and his casket sat in that same parlor, long lines formed in the street, people waiting patiently in the heat of the sun, waiting for a chance to say goodbye to Doctor Wood.

History drives me into a fury, the news of white people especially, the madness reported on television, but I have never apologized for my name.

Only a broken man would ever deny his grandfather, especially one such as this man.

But imagine the trouble this man caused his Methodist parents when he announced that he'd fallen in love with this dark-eyed, vivacious little savage girl. Worse yet, she wouldn't marry him unless he gave up his religion and took on hers – an ancient religion full of symbolism, mystical experiences, chanting, the rituals of cannibalism.

If a man is religious about his religion (and apparently my grand-dad was), then he can't go switching on command. There's the whole business of conversion. He knew about Saint Paul on the road to Damascus. He knew that conversion strikes you suddenly and involuntarily, like a bolt of lightning. Or else it grows on you slowly, like warts. I think my grand-dad argued for the "let's get together and see what happens" approach.

She told him to come back when he'd converted. She'd give him six months.

He took five and a half.

And thus the tribal influence came to topple the Methodist, both in Doctor Wood's heart and in mine.

What kind of people were my grandmother's people?

They were islanders who had crossed the wild sea to settle a lush, green, snake-free paradise somewhere around 800 B.C.

They never developed a civilization, never knew what that meant until civilization was forced upon them in the 18th century. They walked on paths, not streets; their lives were organized around the extended family. They had no politics, no state, no central government. They never built a town.

They fought among themselves to secure or expand group-held territory. Occasionally a strong man would arise who would dominate a large realm, even the whole island for a time. They fought recklessly, naked and screaming. Legends say that their warriors could make incredible leaps, could even jump up onto spears in flight, would fall into monstrous battle furies that have been described as "warp-spasms."

A special class of priest-poets, both men and women, kept alive the traditions, histories, and genealogies of this culture. These bards knew magic and practiced medicine. They moved freely from place to place, welcome wherever they traveled.

Most importantly, my grandmother's people loved place. They lived free, casual lives under the open sky. Their songs are filled with a celebration of the rain, the beasts, lovemaking, the small details of human experience.

They believed that the gods themselves dwelt on the Earth. If one of these people felt it was time to go to Heaven, then he or she would get into a boat and paddle across the open sea, because Heaven was on Earth, just over the horizon.

They accepted Christianity without shedding a drop of blood

(although a deadly plague that killed half of their people moti-
vated their willingness to accept the European God). They
resisted the advancement of English-speaking culture until they
could resist no more. Eventually, their native tongue was banned
from the schools of their own land. Today, although street signs
preserve the old names and books preserve the grammar, few
people speak that language in everyday conversation.

Now these people appear to be civilized. When I'm filling
out a governmental form and I'm asked to check boxes to iden-
tify my ethnic background, I never see a box that describes my
grandmother's people – and, in fact, my people. These people
are assumed to have passed from the Earth.

My grandmother was a Celt.

She, like the majority of my ancestors, was Irish. And by the
way that word "Celt" is pronounced with a hard "K" sound, not
like that band of has-been basketball players from Boston with
their "Seltic," a deliberate British mispronunciation that makes
my blood boil and then I feel a warp-spasm coming on.

Most of all, don't ever call me a "haole."

My people have been insulted, shot, starved, driven into
exile, beaten into submission, scattered across the planet. If you
ever hear an Irishman say "the luck of the Irish," you'll know
how deeply ironic, even sarcastic that phrase can be.

And yet, I once had the pleasure to stand in front of a group
of 300 people on St. Patrick's Day and ask everyone with even
a drop of Irish blood to raise a hand. Two hundred and seven-
ty-eight hands went up.

You see, the Irish are good for something.

So on March 17 you can be sure I'll be lifting a glass of
whiskey to the old folks. Come join me, and then we can have
a long talk about cultural oppression, about sovereignty, about
the extinction of cultures.

An article in the paper recently was telling that human languages are dying off, becoming extinct just like so many plants

and animals. Like it or not, we're living in a time when variety is being sacrificed for uniformity.

They say that 20 to 50 percent of the world's languages even now are no longer learned by the children; these languages are "the living dead." Of the world's 6,000 languages, only 600 are assured of survival 100 years from now.

The Celts have had the lead over so many other cultures and languages in this dying game. Or is it, really, a dying game?

Can anything this strong and good truly pass from the world?

When I lift my glass on the 17th, I'm going to say no. I don't speak the Celtic tongue, live in a crannog, raise cattle, nor when I want to die will I row my way to Tir na Nog in a coracle.

But I have a Celtic hand, and through it rushes the blood of the Sullivans and the Devlins – mingled with other mongrel bloods, and the mix is a good mix. I'm better and stronger for the mix. I'm an alloy of toughness. I have the mind and mouth of a druid, made wiser by my ancestors' vaster experience.

You can say as much about yourself, in your own way, no doubt.

And when the wind stirs the thick grasses here where I live, and the sudden rains come blowing and clothing my house and this land and all those about me – why, I'm telling you, I look out at this place with eyes that are older than my own eyes.

I could swear I'm right back where I belong.

For thanks, I give you a hole in the ground

Tomorrow I'll clean out the imu pit, make sure I still have enough unfractured rocks for another good firing.

Tomorrow is the day before Thanksgiving.

I'll finish cutting up the kiawe logs I brought in last weekend.

To get those logs, we took a two-day scramble around East Maui, and we didn't get back home till the first edge of dawn Monday. We were driving back on the Hana road in the cloud-lit, fading moonlight (or was it queerly early dawn?) with a can of warm Mountain Dew between us and a Thelonius Monk tape turned down low.

It's imu time.

My cooking utensils include a chain saw and a contractor's-size wheelbarrow.

I snapped a shovel handle the other day. Two Ha'iku winters is about all a shovel can take before the wooden handle turns to chalk. So, as odd as it sounds, I've got to buy a new shovel so I can cook the holiday turkey.

After all, I'm cooking a feast for a small tribe.

I'm going to cook a turkey and a leg of lamb, and I'm going to cook them in the style of this land and of its people. (If you're a vegetarian, you'll have to forgive me for talking so bluntly about meat.) If my small tribe were larger, I'd gladly put even MORE meat in my imu. I'd prefer to cook meat that I've raised or hunted myself, but that won't be the case this year. Instead, I pay Foodland to raise or hunt for me. Maybe next year I'll achieve the perfect relationship to my food.

Once again this year, I'm cooking thanksgiving in a fiery hole that shouts to the sky.

Once again this year, I'm going to make the Pilgrims of Plymouth Rock run aground in Polynesia. Once again, The Great White Figureheads will have to stop staring into the heavens and turn to look instead at a pit in the earth.

The Pilgrims' prayer from the pit: *Out from the depths I cry unto You, O Lord. Let my prayer be acceptable in Thy sight.* May the fire rise true, may the wood burn all the way across, may the food cook thoroughly, may the tribe be fed. May the party be loud and embarrassingly uninhibited.

That pit, its walls darkened and maybe even glazed with the heat of earlier firings, still holds the clean, black, many-pitted, remembering stones. Those stones – round, black, glistening wet, smoky smelling – have sat together waiting under a board in the dark. For months they've mumbled together down there like forgotten gods, unvisited except by occasional large insects or spiders. They're ready to glow red-hot again in my purposeful volcano.

Thursday at sunrise I'll stack the dry kiawe and flammables in the imu, building them up around an eight-foot rod that prods vertically out from the base of the pit. The rod will hold itself like a thumb stuck right into the core of the future fire.

Then I'll skin the carefully-built woodstack with a thick shell made of those black stones. Then I'll yank the rod out from the pile center.

For a minute, that open shaft will swallow the power of the zenith straight down. Then the fire will go in.

A fat plume of harmless smoke will surge up into the turbulent Haʻiku sky. And then a great fire will be held in the pit there, contained by earth and stone. I always imagine the fire going straight into the heart of Pele's mountain.

After that, we wait for the stones to sink into the ashes of the spent kiawe. We gather plants from the land around the imu pit. Only thirty feet away, banana stalks are beaten and broken open like the ingredients in some enormous stir-fry. When the moment is right, thicknesses of juicy stems are heaped, steaming, down in the pit over the red-hots.

Women bring forth green baskets of feasting, the food woven and swaddled in leaves. These are set down like pearls into the rising furnace. The top of the heap is then overheaped with more plants, then with narrowing screens of fabric, then the whole fervent oven is totally scarfed in dirt.

Now the feast is a complete secret.

We spend at least half an hour watching for smoke vents – leaks – which the small tribe takes turns attacking with spadefuls of earthy smother. Even an hour or two later people are still saying that they see some smoke coming from the imu. These people are committed to the imu.

The imu is the center of a universe that makes sense to me, and for that I give my utmost thanks. This essay is my thanksgiving shout, my animal/spiritual howl of happiness, delivered without a trace of my usual irony, no trick, no fooling.

The imu ties me to the world; it ties me in every direction. Its stones tie me to the heat of the earth, and, as the smoke rises, that same heat ties me to the tumbling heavens. My tribe converges on this single spot, knitting its intentions together through many small orchestrated chores. Then the pit is opened; the good food is passed from hand to hand.

Eating is never the important point of a feast like this. Eating is humdrum and private and, in the end, nothing but crap. The doing is everything. The tying-together.

Let the food spill forth. Taste a little, then give it all away. Let no one go hungry! Let nothing go to waste! We are here to act out the rituals of connectedness: Human bound to Earth and to Sky and to Tribe, Human fully alive in the intricating Now....

And I'm forgetting the Past, too, and that's not right, for the imu ties me even tighter to the past than it does to the present.

I have many histories, but my most important history is the history of the land that feeds me, the land I care for. On Thursday dawn, as I set fire to the stones and the earth, I will lift my heart in gratitude to the Hawaiians, who have taught me how to live here. I have been a slow, but willing, student.

Before I began writing this article, I intended to celebrate my freedom – the fact that I can shut my gate on the world and spend whole days far from the choked streets of Kahului, the clutter of Kihei, the high-rise insults of Honolulu.

I intended to celebrate the fact that Long's Drugs is still 30 minutes away, not ten, that Kmart is way, way down there, that all supermarkets are inconveniently far away. So far, my life is still good, still as I would choose it.

But why should I be so profane, when this may be my last moment under this moist sky, tonight's rain my last wetting, this shovelful of earth my final purposeful act?

Stone, fire, stem, flesh. These are my sacraments. A spadeful of earth lifted into the heavens. The imu ties me and lashes me into place.

God's belly button. The piko of my life.

And I am happy to be here, at the center of everything.

ⓑ

GLOSSARY

'A'a - Rough-style lava rock, common on Maui. Giant cheese grater type ground.

A&B - Alexander & Baldwin, Incorporated, the Maui firm (est. 1869) generally considered responsible for everything — for Hurricane Iniki, for World War II, for the tidal wave of 1946, for every car accident, extraterrestrial sighting, sunburn, and unspayed pet on this island for the past 100 years.

Ahi - The yellowfin tuna, a big fish often spotted hanging around in sushi bars.

Aloha - Kindest regards; good vibes. The earnest desire to be a fine person.

Auwe! - oh no!

Brah - term of address suitable if one or more of the following conditions apply: 1) man is wearing rubber slippers; 2) man has pig carcass tied to hood of truck; 3) boy; 4) man is standing in front of marijuana field with a shotgun.

Captain James Cook - William Shatner's role model. An industrious farmboy from Yorkshire England who became one of Western history's greatest maritime explorers. Hawai'i's first known tourist, he sailed past Maui's North Shore in 1779 so as not to miss his rendezvous with death in a Big Island brawl.

Chicken skin - Horripilation.

Choke - (Pidgin English) A large amount of. (Q: "How much stuffs you get already?" A: "Choke! Only planny! Like try?"

Downhill bikers - Those who ride bicycles from Haleakala Crater (10,031 feet elevation) to the sea, a 35 mile trip which takes about 10 minutes if you go for it and all day if you pay $100 and get in an incompetent lineup with other tourists who, like you, are all wearing pink football helmets.

Haole - Whitey; honky; round-eyed imperialist devil, destroyer of all that is sacred. (See "A&B".)

Heiau - Large lava-rock platforms erected by the old Hawaiians as sacred sites, temple compounds, seats of authority.

Hippie - Any "haole" (q.v.) who is A) not employed by A&B, and B) not a retiree.

Ho'opono - to correct; to behave correctly.

Imu - traditional Hawaiian earth oven: hot-rock underground cooking with banana and ti leaf steam, suitable for feeding tribes.

Ka'ahumanu - Hawaiian queen (1777 - 1832) who governed the islands for 13 years, during which time she tossed out the entire system of Hawaiian faith and government and imposed missionary-twisted, Western-style thinking. In doing so, she slowed down the extinction of her own culture. As a weird gesture of thanks, Maui has put her name on its largest shopping mall.

Kaho'olawe - An island in Maui County formerly dedicated to the Hawaiian god Kanaloa, the former home of a school for the heroic science of Polynesian open-sea navigation. In the early 1940s, the U.S. military decided that the island was a piece of junk. They seized it and then dropped bombs on it for 50 years. After Hawaiian citizens began dying in protest of this stupidity, the military withdrew and left behind its litter of 1,200 tons of scrap and 6,000 unexploded bombs. Now the Republican-led federal government is whining about cleaning up its own mess.

Kahuna - Any respected Hawaiian authority with specialized training in a field vital to the survival of culture. A priest/doctor/poet/craftsperson/druid.

Kamehameha - The Hawaiian strongman (1753 - 1819) who took advantage of post-Captain-Cook chaos to seize control of the entire island chain for the first time in its history. When he died in 1819, everything fell apart. The first boatload of missionaries arrived one year later.

Kapa - or "tapa cloth." Hawaiian fabric, made by laboriously pounding, layering, and softening certain kinds of tree bark, and then stamping and dyeing designs.

Kapu - Forbidden; a formal announcement that something is off-limits or forbidden. (The Tahitian version of this word: taboo.) The rules that governed ancient Hawaiian life are called, collectively, "the kapu system."

Kau'iki Head - A prominent landmark that forms the right arm of Hana Bay, a large pu'u (cinder cone hill) now overgrown with ironwood trees.

Kiawe - A thorny hardwood tree, introduced to Hawai'i in the 1840s, which provides the firewood preferred for the imu. Also known as mesquite.

Kim chee - Spicy, stinky Korean pickled cabbage. Best if you can figure out how to eat it without ever opening the jar indoors.

Lahainaluna - District on the uphill side of Lahaina, Maui, home of the oldest American school west of the Rockies. The old printing house here produced Bibles, textbooks, paper money, each one a nail in the coffin of traditional island culture.

Liberty House - Hawai'i's answer to Nieman-Marcus, a high-end department store, the foundation tenant of Maui's Ka'ahumanu Shopping Center.

Limu - Seaweed, especially if you eat it.

Local - The opposite of haole (q.v.), which is all extremely simple except when you run into a local who isn't very local or a haole who is.

Lo'i - A traditional taro-growing patch that's constantly flooded and refreshed with mountain water.

Maile - A native forest vine with subtly pungent foliage. Getting a maile lei, made by stripping the leaves and bark and winding them together, is a sure sign that someone thinks you're pretty darn great.

Maka'ainana - The common people; the tribe. Literally, the "eyes of the land." David Malo in *Hawaiian Antiquities*: "The commoners were the most numerous class of people in the nation, and were known as the ma-ka-aina-na; another name by which they were called was hu. (Hu, to swell, multiply, increase like yeast.)" Jesus in *Luke*: "Blest are you poor; the reign of God is yours."

Makahiki - David Malo: "The Makahiki was a time when men, women and chiefs rested and abstained from all work, either on the farm or elsewhere." This fall festival season was dedicated to the god Lono; the fact that Captain Cook arrived in the midst of a Makahiki celebration bearing all the distinctive marks of the god Lono himself will always remain one of the weirdest ironies of the colonial era.

Makai - See Mauka/makai.

Makani - Wind, breeze; gas in the stomach.

Makapiapia - Boogers in the eyes.

Malama - To care for, preserve.

Malihini - Stranger, newcomer, foreigner; guest. Handy and Pukui in *The Polynesian Family System in Ka'u Hawai'i*: "...she was kama'aina, for she was the native "daughter of the land" (kama'aina) who took the strangers (malihini) to see places of interest."

Malo - The man's loincloth. Handy and Pukui: "In explaining near kinship a kupuna would say, Nou ka malo, nana e hume; nona ka malo, nau e hume, or 'Your malo he can wear; his malo you can wear.'"

David Malo - An early Maui historian and native Hawaiian scholar, teacher, and statesman who graduated from Lahainaluna School in 1835 at the age of 42. Malo helped draft the first Hawaiian declaration of rights and constitution, and he wrote an important record of traditional Hawaiian practices, *Hawaiian Antiquities.* Thinking ahead to the Maui we now inhabit, he wrote: "If a big wave comes in, large and unfamiliar fishes will come from the dark ocean, and when they see the small fishes of the shallows they will eat them up."

Mana - Divine power, which is resident in rocks, bones, fingernail clippings, and all things of this divine world.

Maui Land & Pine - Maui Land & Pineapple Company. (See A&B.)

Mauka/makai - Basic directions for island-living people in Hawai'i. "Ma-uka" means literally "toward the mountain." "Ma-kai" means "toward the ocean." Mainland-style directions: "Take Highway 360 east to the corner of Kalo Road and turn right." Maui-style directions: "Go Hana. Bymby going check out mile marker thirty-one. Get one street there. Go mauka."

MEO bus - This island has no public transportation system, but Maui Economic Opportunity, Inc., a county-wide social service organization, has little buses that will pick you up and drop you off. The old folks are hip to this. The young prefer illegal hitch-hiking, with the risk of getting shoved and insulted by an irritable cop.

Missionary - Uninvited know-it-all. "Moral indignation is jealousy with a halo." - H.G. Wells.

Moke - An unflattering group label for any tough local guy.

Musubi - A ball of rice that you can carry around till you feel like eating it. Generally served with a plank of fried Spam on top, the whole package wrapped in nori, edible black seaweed.

Ni'ihau - A small, mysterious Hawaiian island inhabited only by Hawaiians. No one's ever been there, no one ever talks about it, and I'm sorry I even mentioned it.

'Oha - After you harvest the taro, you take the 'oha − the living stem with the top of the root − and replant it. That's continuity. That's culture.

'Ohana - All the 'oha together: the family, the big family, the tribe.

Okole - Rear end; derriere.

Opihi - A popular wild food, raw or cooked. Sea snails. Pop 'em off the rocks down where the waves are crashing.

'O'o - Digging stick.

Piko - Belly button. Omphalos. Center of the universe.

Poi - Purple, nutritious goo made by pounding steamed taro root. The bread and butter of old Hawai'i.

Poi dog - The kind suitable for ancient Hawaiian barbecues; fattened up all soft and tender because they've been eating poi.

Pono - Goodness, moral rectitude; excellence.

Pukalani bypass - A recently-completed high-speed Upcountry thoroughfare. It replaces the inconvenience of driving slowly through the town of Pukalani with the modern convenience of smashing into one another at 60 miles per hour.

Pu'u - Cinder cone; Small rounded hill formed by the blowing-out of billions of small pieces of fluffy lava. A typical feature of the volcanic rift zones.

Sky-Hoist - A ridiculous fabrication of one writer's imagination. For season tickets, send $200 to this address.

Sovereignty - The enduring fantasy that the Hawaiians will once again govern these islands, an extremely popular notion with non-Hawaiians.

Statehood - The official contract, signed in 1959, requiring Hawai'i to build Kmarts, condominiums, munitions dumps, Star Wars tracking stations, automated gas station/mini-marts, and in general to behave just as stupidly as the United States of America.

Stink-eye - The vicious, murderous stare of death.

Taro (kalo) - *Colocasia esculenta*, a typical marsh plant bearing a short underground corm in which starch is stored, originated in the East Indies and was carried by the Polynesians throughout their Pacific migrations.

Ti (ki) - Another one of those plants, like taro, that the Polynesians brought with them when they traveled, a kind of *Dracaena* bush that makes everyone happy with its big, cool, gladsome leaves that you can wear if you like. (No longer suitable as everyday attire.)

Tilapia - A fish that thrives in brackish water, mud puddles, ditches, bogs, murky ponds, and discarded saucepans.

Tutu - Grandma; grandma-like person.

Upcountry - The mountain country of East Maui, a loose geographical term with no precise boundaries, a mental state with no precise definition.